Field Guide to the
Normal Newborn

W9-BZR-137

Field Guide to the Normal Newborn

Gary A. Emmett, M.D., F.A.A.P.
Clinical Assistant Professor and
Director of General Pediatrics
Thomas Jefferson University
Philadelphia, Pennsylvania

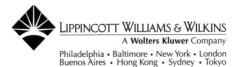

LIPPINCOTT WILLIAMS & WILKINS
A **Wolters Kluwer** Company

Philadelphia • Baltimore • New York • London
Buenos Aires • Hong Kong • Sydney • Tokyo

Acquisitions Editor: Timothy Hiscock
Developmental Editor: Lisa Consoli
Production Editor: Jeff Somers
Manufacturing Manager: Ben Rivera
Cover Designer: Patricia Gast
Compositor: TechBooks
Printer: RR Donnelley

© **2004 by LIPPINCOTT WILLIAMS & WILKINS**
530 Walnut Street
Philadelphia, PA 19106 USA
LWW.com

Printed in the USA

Library of Congress Cataloging-in-Publication Data

Emmett, Gary A.
  Field guide to the normal newborn / Gary A. Emmett.
    p. ; cm.
  Includes bibliographical references and index.
  ISBN 0-7817-2877-0 (pbk.)
  1. Neonatology. I. Title.
  [DNLM: 1. Perinatal Care—methods. 2. Infant Care—methods. 3. Infant, Newborn, Diseases. 4. Neonatal Screening. WQ 210 E54f 2004]
RJ251.E46 2004
618.92′01—dc22

                                                                2004008104

Care has been taken to confirm the accuracy of the information presented and to describe generally accepted practices. However, the authors, editor, and publisher are not responsible for errors or omissions or for any consequences from application of the information in this book and make no warranty, expressed or implied, with respect to the currency, completeness, or accuracy of the contents of the publication. Application of this information in a particular situation remains the professional responsibility of the practitioner.

The authors, editor, and publisher have exerted every effort to ensure that drug selection and dosage set forth in this text are in accordance with current recommendations and practice at the time of publication. However, in view of ongoing research, changes in government regulations, and the constant flow of information relating to drug therapy and drug reactions, the reader is urged to check the package insert for each drug for any change in indications and dosage and for added warnings and precautions. This is particularly important when the recommended agent is a new or infrequently employed drug.

Some drugs and medical devices presented in this publication have Food and Drug Administration (FDA) clearance for limited use in restricted research settings. It is the responsibility of the health care provider to ascertain the FDA status of each drug or device planned for use in their clinical practice.

                                                10 9 8 7 6 5 4 3 2 1

Preface

The Field Guide to the Normal Newborn is a short text to introduce the management of the well, full-term or almost full-term newborn who is in the well baby nursery. Being in the well nursery does not necessarily make you a well child. In general, these chapters deal with the everyday problems and quandaries that will arise in the course of having a new infant go through transition, bond with his mother, and to learn to be nourished by her and others. To facilitate the rapid acquisition of usable information, many chapters will contain an algorithm (decision tree) that will quickly take the practitioner to the solution of the immediate problem. The chapter contains more detailed information about the nature of the specific problem and its solution. At the end of the chapter, you will see "suggested readings." Some of this material will be online, all of it will be easily obtainable. In chapters that concern physical examinations that are not related to specific diagnostics or treatment dilemmas, there will be no introductory algorithm.

This book is a work in progress. If you have any ideas on how to improve the book, particularly in regards to chapters that present information in innovative manners (for example Table 21.1 Maternal Diseases Effecting Neonates), please contact me at gemmett@nemours.org.

Acknowledgments

I would like to thank all the people who provided me with editorial assistance: my daughters, Gillian, Ariel, and Ilana Emmett; my son Isaac Emmett; and Daniel Mozes. I would also like to thank all of the physicians who contributed to this book. Finally I would like to thank Tim Hiscock who tolerated my endless delays so well.

Contents

Part IV: After Discharge

Appendices

Contributing Authors

Linda M. Asta, M.D. *Clinical Assistant Professor, Department of Pediatrics, University of California at San Francisco, San Francisco, California; Chair, Department of Pediatrics, John Muir Medical Center, Walnut Creek, California*

Mae Coleman, M.D. *Neonatal Associates of Jacksonville, Jacksonville, Florida*

Jay Goldberg, M.D. *Clinical Assistant Professor, Department of Obstetrics and Gynecology, Jefferson Medical College, Philadelphia, Pennsylvania*

Erika B. Johnston, M.D. *Second Year Resident, Department of Obstetrics and Gynecology, Jefferson Medical College, Philadelphia, Pennsylvania*

Sue Jue, M.D. *Louisiana State University Health Sciences Center at Shreveport, Shreveport, Louisiana*

J. Lindsey Lane, M.D. *Associate Professor of Pediatrics, Department of Pediatrics, Thomas Jefferson University, Philadelphia, Pennsylvania*

William G. McNett, M.D. *Clinical Instructor, Department of Pediatrics, Thomas Jefferson University, Philadelphia, Pennsylvania*

Linda D. Meloy, M.D. *Clinical Associate Professor of Pediatrics, Virginia Commonwealth University, Richmond, Virginia*

John Mark Olsson, M.D. *Associate Professor, Department of Pediatrics, Brody School of Medicine, East Carolina University, Greenville, North Carolina*

Budd N. Shenkin, M.D, M.A.P.A. *President, Bayside Medical Group, Oakland, California*

Nicholas Slamon, M.D. *Resident in Pediatrics, Thomas Jefferson University/duPont Pediatric Residency, Philadelphia, Pennsylvania*

William B. Stephenson, M.D. *General Pediatrician, Department of Pediatrics, Penobscot Bay Medical Center, Rockport, Maine*

Judith Anne Turow, M.D. *Clinical Assistant Professor of Pediatrics, Department of Pediatrics, Thomas Jefferson University, Philadelphia, Pennsylvania*

Part I

Delivery Room and Before

CHAPTER 1

The Prenatal Visit

Lisa M. Asta

First impressions do count.

The practitioner can use the prenatal visit to improve the care of the new baby. Figure 1.1 guides the practitioner through the prenatal appointment, and Table 1.1 lists individual items that the practitioner should discuss with the parents.

During the prenatal visit, expectant parents and the practitioner inaugurate a collaborative relationship that can last through a child's college years. This optional appointment, which can take many forms, allows participants to ask questions, share information, and learn about each other. The practitioner can help parents move smoothly through the first few weeks of their new baby's life with relevant information on child health and safety.

Parents may schedule the prenatal appointment at any time during the pregnancy, but because premature birth can occur, it should ideally take place early in the third trimester. Obstetricians often encourage expectant parents to schedule an introductory visit with the child's practitioner. In that way, the primary care practitioner can be available should there be prenatal issues (for example, a chromosomal abnormality or a structural abnormality such as congenital heart disease). Obstetricians provide families with local practitioners' names and phone numbers.

Some parents simply call a practice, ask if they are taking new patients, and select that practice after a brief discussion with the office staff. Many practices prepare written information that reviews office hours, after-hours care, insurance, fees, and other pertinent information. This material should be mailed to prospective parents, or the pamphlets can be provided to families when they arrive for their prenatal appointment.

Face-to-face prenatal appointments can vary in length, with a maximum of 45 minutes allowed by the practitioner. We suggest they be done outside of patient-care hours so that they can be somewhat open-ended. Some parents just want to be able to recognize the face that they will next see in a much more stressful atmosphere; these visits can take only 10 minutes. Some come with pages of questions, and it is wise in this case to say that the session must end by a fixed time stated at the very beginning of the interview. Most practices do not charge for the prenatal visit; some insurances will pay for this visit, however, and local market conditions determine whether a charge can be assessed.

Begin with a basic history of the family and the course of the pregnancy. Table 1.2 provides guidelines.

Asking parents if they have specific questions can be an excellent, open-ended way to help organize and direct the meeting. Parents often ask about doctors' credentials, hospital affiliations, hours, telephone

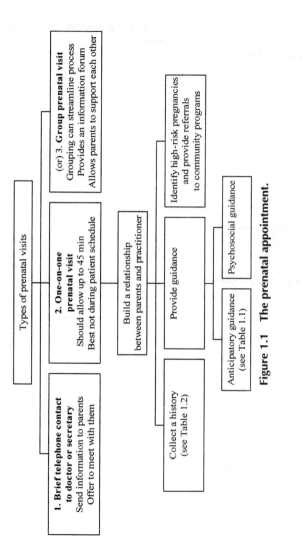

Figure 1.1   The prenatal appointment.

Table 1.1 Anticipatory guidance

Adjust hot water	Temperature $<120°$F
Baby equipment	Need car seat, crib, seat for house "The only soft thing your baby needs is you"
"Back to sleep"	Child must sleep on back until able to turn over
Car seat safety	Must have car seat prior to birth and know how to install it properly
Childbirth class	Wonderful way to learn about birth and feeding
Crib safety	Discuss bassinets, cribs, use of toys, bumpers, and pillows
Drugs, alcohol	Dangers pre- and postnatally
HIV testing	If positive, usually can prevent transmission to baby
Infant CPR class	Introduction that increases feeling of safety
No baby walkers	May cause serious accidents
No bottle in bed	Can lead to choking, ear infections, and later to cavities
Smoke detectors	Also fire and carbon dioxide detectors
Smoke-free environment	To lead to eventual smoking cessation
Thermometers	Must learn how to use in hospital

advice, and after-hours care. They may also ask about the practice's philosophy regarding breast-feeding, circumcision, immunizations, and antibiotic use. Many practitioners simply answer all of these questions in a short introduction of 2 to 5 minutes to start, as detailed in Table 1.3. Periodic review of the sample interview questions published in parenting books and magazines can keep the practitioner's interviewing technique fresh.

Most parents, however, do not come with prepared questions, and a more pediatrician-directed approach is required. Begin building the relationship by encouraging fathers and extended family to participate in the child's health care. Invite grandparents, great aunts, and significant adults to come to appointments. Family members often offer advice on everything from burping to bike helmets, and an open dialog across generations builds mutual respect and enhances a collaborative relationship.

Practitioners can collect family-specific information by interviewing the parents or having them complete a brief registration sheet. Explore whether the family is prepared to deal with the stress of the new baby on the household, including whether arrangements have

Table 1.2   History at prenatal interview

Course of pregnancy	• EDC, gravida • Chronic illnesses • Alcohol/street drug use • Dehydration/vomiting • Medications/herbs • Allergies • Lupus	• Hospitalizations • Sugar elevation • BP elevation • Blood type/antibodies	• Positive test(s) for: • Hepatitis B or C • Group B streptococcus • Chlamydia/gonorrhea • Herpes simplex • Syphilis • HIV
Family history	• Mother • Father • Siblings • Age, health, profession for each	• Structure of household • Is anyone in the home immune-suppressed?	• Asthma/eczema/allergies • Bleeding disorders • Congenital heart defect • Early death (<age 50) • Seizures • Infections, esp. TB
Household	• Smoking • Smoke/fire/CO alarms	• Pets • Lead	• Guns • Fluoride in water
Social history	• Do cultural or religious beliefs limit medical care for the infant?	• Is there use or abuse of illicit or licit drugs?	• Is there a history of physical or sexual abuse in house?
Postpartum plans	• Breast- or bottle-feeding	• Short- and long-term caretaker plans	• Is house ready for the new baby?

Table 1.3   Practitioner short self-presentation

Practice rules and hours	Include night and weekend coverage System of telephone advice
Practitioner's credentials	Include hospital affiliations
Feeding	Support breast-feeding
Circumcision	Are you for it, against it, neutral? Is it done by you or the obstetrician?
Immunizations	Visits, shots, especially the first year
Treatment philosophy	Especially antibiotic use

been made for outside child care. To find questions that provide insight into the family unit, see Table 1.2 (social history). Ask only social questions that the practitioner is willing to follow up.

Most new parents are convinced that they will be nervous. Often the simple reassurance that everyone is a nervous new parent at first will ease this anxiety. Pediatricians may also encourage parents to attend baby-care classes and may recommend simple, readable books on child care. *Caring for Your Baby and Young Child* from the American Academy of Pediatrics is one good resource.

The prenatal appointment is an excellent time to provide anticipatory guidance. New parents are often highly motivated to do things right. Published guidelines from the American Academy of Pediatrics, Bright Futures, and Guidelines for Health Supervision provide exhaustive topics for discussion. The sensitive pediatrician will optimize the prenatal visit by answering parents' questions and tailoring their anticipatory guidance. In this manner, the participants will learn about each other and decide if their chemistry is right.

Ask parents whether they are planning to breast-feed or bottle-feed, and discuss the advantages of breast-feeding. Review the support services nursing mothers can obtain from the pediatrician and lactation professionals. Teach parents always to put the baby to sleep on the back to reduce the risk of sudden infant death syndrome (SIDS). Discuss the risks of sleeping with the infant.

Many parents have questions about circumcision. Some parents come to the appointment having already decided; others ask about the pros and cons of the procedure. Parents like to know where and when the procedure will be done. Be prepared to discuss the risks and benefits and the use of anesthesia.

Use Table 1.1 for other important topics in anticipatory guidance. Encourage parents to keep all their appointments with the obstetrician and to attend childbirth, child care, and CPR classes. Review the schedule for well visits and immunizations.

Psychosocial guidance can be woven throughout the previous discussions. Help parents anticipate the change in family relationships. Encourage them to share infant care, use the support system of family and friends, and prepare siblings. Acknowledge the fatigue and depression that may accompany a new baby. Remind parents, who may have extremely high expectations for themselves and their baby, that it is okay not to meet all of them.

Practitioners learn a great deal about their future patient at the prenatal visit. Take notes (this is required if you plan to charge a fee and is good practice at all times). High-risk pregnancies and difficult social situations may warrant referrals to community resources (WIC, food stamps, housing, counseling, and alcohol and substance abuse programs), breast-feeding support, parenting classes, or new parents groups. Be prepared to access a social work source from the hospital or your practice who can devote more time and expertise to these difficult areas.

The prenatal appointment starts a relationship with a family, promotes the health of a new child, and is an excellent opportunity for promotion of a medical practice.

SUGGESTED READINGS

American Academy of Pediatrics, Committee on Psychosocial Aspects of Child and Family Health. The prenatal visit. *Pediatrics* 2001;108:1456–1458.

Bright Futures Project: National Center for Education in Maternal and Child Health. *Bright futures: guidelines for health supervision of infants, children, and adolescents.* 1998. <www.brightfutures.org>

Dershewitz R. Prenatal anticipatory guidance. *Clin Perinatol* 1985;12: 343–353.

Shelov SP, Hanneman RE. *The American Academy of Pediatrics: caring for your baby and young child: birth to age 5.* New York: Bantam Books, 1998.

The Delivery Room

Mae M. Coleman

The ability to successfully resuscitate a newborn is often the entryway to a successful community practice of pediatrics.

Although only a small percentage of infants need prolonged resuscitative efforts, it is difficult to predict which infants will need intervention. Therefore, the infant resuscitator attends many deliveries where he or she is not needed. What is important is that the resuscitator is always ready for all likely eventualities. This neonatal resuscitation protocol will help transition the infant to successful extrauterine life. See Figs. 2.1 and 2.2 and Tables 2.1 and 2.2.

Apgar scoring (Table 2.3) is a relatively objective score that correlates with the state of an infant at given times after birth. This score is assigned at 1 and 5 minutes for well babies and every 2 minutes thereafter if the child is not stable (until a score of 7 or greater is achieved). The Apgar score should not be used as an indicator to begin resuscitation in a depressed infant, but inability to reach a score of 8 implies that a child needs to be placed in an observation bed and not a level 1 nursery. Apgar scores of 7 or less after 5 minutes generally indicate a poor transition to extrauterine life, and these infants require further evaluation.

Meconium is the passage of fetal stool, which stains the amniotic fluid and can be aspirated into the infant's mouth and potentially into the infant's airways. If the meconium in the amniotic fluid is thin, special management of this infant is probably not necessary. If the meconium in the amniotic fluid is thick and particulate, it must be cleared from the airway. Table 2.4 lists medications for neonatal resuscitation in the delivery room.

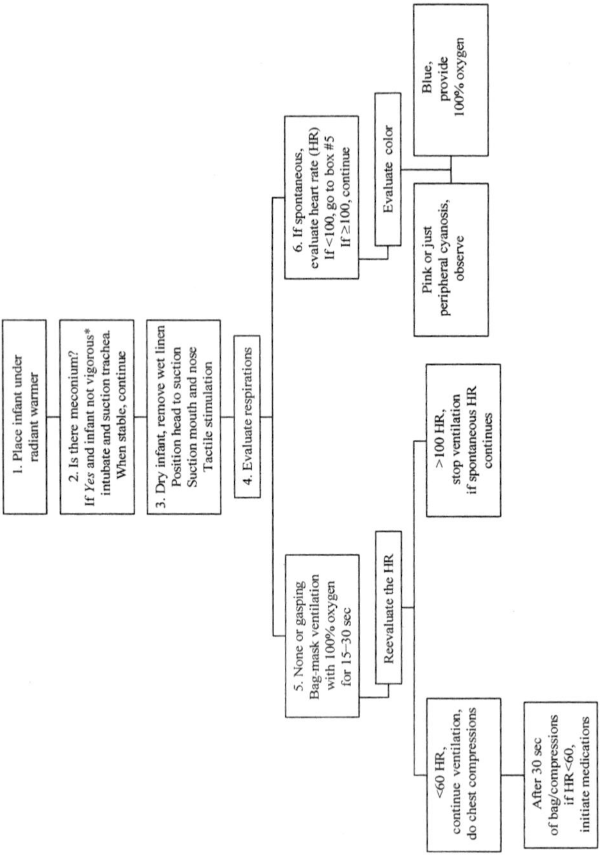

Figure 2.1   Overview of delivery room resuscitation.

* vigorous: strong respiratory efforts, good muscle tone, and a heart rate greater than 100 bpm.

Table 2.1   Standard equipment and supplies for neonatal resuscitation

Suction equipment	Bulb syringe	
	Mechanical suction	
	Suction catheters (6F, 8F, 10F)	
	Feeding tube (8F)	
	Meconium aspirator	
Bag-mask equipment	Neonatal resuscitation bag with pressure gauge	
	Face masks	
	Oral airways	
	Oxygen source and tubing	
	Oxygen flowmeter	
Intubation equipment	Laryngoscope	
	Laryngoscope straight blades (No. 1)	
	Endotracheal tubes (2.5, 3.0, 3.5, 4.0 mm)	
	Stylet	
Other equipment	Alcohol	Syringes (1, 3, 5, 10, 20, 50 mL)
	Stopcock	
	Stethoscope	Needles (25, 21, 18 gauge)
	Gloves	
	Scissors	Umbilical artery catheterization tray with umbilical tape
	Adhesive tape	
		Umbilical catheters (3.5, 5 F)
		Radiant warmer

Table 2.2   Initiation of neonatal resuscitation

Steps to a Successful Transition	
Thermal management	Place infant in preheated radiant warmer
	Dry infant with a warm towel
	Remove wet blankets
Airway clearance	Suction mouth first with bulb syringe
	Suction nose gently with bulb syringe
Tactile stimulation	If drying and suctioning fail, slap soles of newborn's feet or rub back

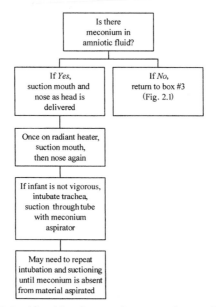

Figure 2.2   Algorithm for treating meconium at delivery.

Table 2.3   Apgar score

Parameter	0	1	2
Heart rate	Absent	<100 beats per minute (bpm)	>100 bpm
Respiratory effort	Absent	Slow, irregular	Good, crying
Muscle tone	Flaccid	Some flexion	Active motion of extremities
Reflex irritability	No response	Grimace	Vigorous cry
Color	Completely pale or cyanotic	Peripheral cyanosis	Completely pink

Table 2.4   Medications for neonatal resuscitation in the delivery room

Medication	Concentration	Preparation	Dosage/Route	Precautions
Epinephrine	1:10000	1 mL	0.1–0.3 mL/kg IV or ET	Give rapidly Dilute with 1–2 mL sterile saline
Volume expanders	Whole blood Normal saline Ringer's lactate	40 mL	10 mL/kg IV, IO	Give over 5 to 10 min
Sodium bicarbonate	0.5 mEq/mL (4.2% solution)	10 mL	2 mEq/kg IV	Give slowly over at least 2 min Give only if ventilated
Naloxone	0.4 mg/mL	1 mL	0.1 mg/kg (0.25 mL/kg) IV, ET, IM, SQ	Give rapidly ET route preferred
	1.0 mg/mL	2 mL	0.1 mg/kg (0.1 mL/kg) IV, ET, IM, SQ	Give rapidly ET route preferred

IV, intravenous; ET, endotracheal; IM, intramuscular; SQ, subcutaneous; IO, intraosseous.

SUGGESTED READING

Bloom RS, Cropley C. *Textbook of neonatal resuscitation.* American Heart Association, 1994.

Fanaroff AA, Martin RJ. *Neonatal-perinatal medicine: diseases of the fetus and infant,* 6th ed. St. Louis, MO: Mosby, 1997.

International Guidelines for Neonatal Resuscitation: An Excerpt from the Guidelines 2000 for Cardiopulmonary Resuscitation and Emergency Cardiovascular Care: International Consensus on Science. *Pediatrics* 2000;106(3).

Kattwinkel J. (Ed) *Textbook of Neonatal Resuscitation, 4th Edition.* American Academy of Pediatrics, 2000.

CHAPTER 3

Stabilization

Mae M. Coleman

Transition is difficult: a few minutes to go from being water breathing to air breathing.

Prevention of heat loss in the delivery room is an important consideration in basic neonatal resuscitation (see Fig. 2.1). In utero, the fetus's core body temperature is warmer than its mother's temperature. The temperature gradient between the newborn and the ambient air (conduction) and between the baby and the relatively cold walls of the delivery room (radiation) expose the newborn to significant cold stress. An infant's large surface area to weight ratio (three times that of the average adult) causes large conductive, radiant, and evaporative heat losses. Being wet and naked only increases heat loss. The infant should be immediately placed onto a preheated radiant warmer after delivery. The skin and scalp should be dried with warm towels, the infant swaddled, and a cap placed on the head. The combination of a warmer and swaddling will maintain the baby's temperature. A natural alternative, if the mother is awake and alert and if the baby is stable, is to dry the baby and then place against the mother's skin with blankets covering baby and mother. The resuscitation of a newborn should not be allowed to interfere with steps toward thermal protection.

SUGGESTED READING

Fanaroff AA, Martin RJ. *Neonatal-perinatal medicine: diseases of the fetus and infant,* 6th ed. St. Louis, MO: Mosby, 1997.

Goldsmith JP, Karotkin EH. *Assisted ventilation of the neonate.* Philadelphia: WB Saunders, 1981.

Halamek LP, Benaron DA, Stevenson DK. Neonatal hypoglycemia, part I: background and definition. *Clin Pediatr* 1997;36:675–680.

Halamek LP, Stevenson DK. Neonatal hypoglycemia, part II: pathophysiology and therapy. *Clin Pediatr* 1998;37:11–16.

Schwartz MW, ed. *Clinical handbook of pediatrics,* 2nd ed. Baltimore: Williams & Wilkins, 1999.

CHAPTER 4

Admission to the Well Nursery

Gary A. Emmett

Close adherence to clinical pathways prevents well nursery babies from harm by reminding the practitioner that sometimes there are ill babies in the well baby nursery.

After birth, a newborn must successfully complete *transition,* the process of rapidly going from an aquatic creature supported entirely by its mother to an air-breathing human being existing independently. If the child is placed in a properly supportive environment, the vast majority of infants greater than 36 weeks of gestation will successfully complete transition within 2 to 8 hours of birth. The admission process to the well nursery is designed to facilitate that transition by providing the appropriate environment to support transition and by detecting when the child is failing to make a proper transition. See Fig. 4.1.

Selecting the appropriate babies in the delivery room to be admitted to the well nursery versus the special care nursery will prevent most transition problems. Although different birth facilities have different capabilities in their well nurseries versus their special care nurseries, see Table 4.1 for a typical list of well nursery admission criteria.

The key to aiding transition is the proper observation of the newborn's vital signs. A standard well baby care-map for vital signs is presented in Table 4.2. The most important vital signs are color, heart rate, respiratory rate, temperature, and hydration state. Table 4.3 demonstrates how to obtain an infant's temperature properly, and Table 4.4 explains how to measure an infant's pulse and respiratory rate correctly. The monitoring of serum glucose levels is often an important addition, especially if transition is not going well.

Height, weight, and head circumference should be recorded as baselines as soon after delivery as possible. These should be plotted against standard forms. (See Chapter 22.) Weight and percentage of weight loss or gain is measured daily in breast-fed babies and at the beginning of the second day of life in bottle-fed babies.

Most newborns are at least peripherally cyanotic immediately after birth. By the time a child is in the well nursery, he or she should be at least centrally pink, and if the child is still cyanotic, the percutaneous partial pressure of oxygen should be measured. Facial suffusion, echymosis of the face usually associated with a nuchal umbilical cord, may give the false impression of cyanosis in a child soon after birth. Causes of persistent cyanosis include respiratory distress, congenital heart disease, hypoglycemia, hypothermia, or failure of transition.

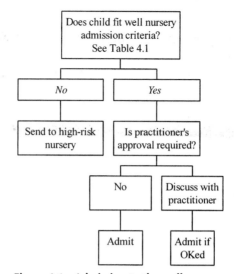

Figure 4.1   Admission to the well nursery.

Heart rate in a newborn should initially be above 100 beats per minute (bpm) and under 180. In larger babies, especially if they are postdates, sleeping heart rates in the 90 to 100 bpm range are acceptable. Causes of abnormal heart rates include the list mentioned previously under color, but also can be produced by maternal disease (lupus), maternal medications (tricyclic antidepressants), and heart conduction defects. In addition, heart failure from whatever cause may result in severe tachycardia.

A newborn can have an initial respiratory rate as high as 90 breaths per minute with no disease found, but rates of 70 or higher are often associated with disease states. All of the diseases and conditions mentioned previously may result in tachypnea. In addition to all the respiratory problems, such as pneumonia, found in older children, newborns also have unique causes of fast breathing. Transient tachypnea of the newborn (TTN) is most commonly found in Caesarean section deliveries and in precipitous deliveries. In TTN, the excess fluid in the chest wall does not get completely squeezed out, and it takes 6 to 24 hours for the child's breathing to return to normal. Diagnosis is made in a tachypnic, but not dyspneic, full-term infant who has a chest X-ray that shows thickening of the lung wall, especially along the fissure between the right upper lobe and the right middle lobe. These children are usually not hypoxic. Supportive care such as an intravenous infusion may be necessary if the child's tachypnea is persistently above 80 and the child is unable to feed otherwise. Myocarditis, pneumothorax, and, more

17

Table 4.1 Admission criteria for the well nursery

May be admitted without practitioner consultation

- Infants ≥2,000 g and ≥36 weeks gestation
- Infants born with an Apgar score ≥0.7 at 5 min
- Infants demonstrating vital signs within normal limits: heart rate 100–180
- Infants showing no signs of respiratory distress

May be admitted after practitioner approval

- Infants for observation/treatment of neonatal abstinence syndrome (NAS)
- Infants being observed for possible sepsis
- Prolonged rupture of membranes (>16 hr)
- Exposure to group B streptococcus not yet requiring treatment
- After complete sepsis work-up in high-risk nursery, as below, even with heparin lock intravenous antibiotics
- Maternal temperature greater than 100.4°F
- Infants with stable blood glucose born to mothers with gestational diabetes
- Infants with blood glucose <50
- Infants with meconium-stained amniotic fluid, even if intubated temporarily in delivery room
- Infants requiring phototherapy for hyperbilirubinemia
- Infants who are delivered outside of hospital who have not been admitted to any other pediatric unit or nursery
- Infants requiring prolonged attendance by neonatology staff (e.g., more than 20 min)
- Infants with weights >4,200 g

seriously, failure to undergo transition may also cause similar problems. Strict observation, avoidance of aspiration by not feeding a child with excess respiratory rates (80 or above), and giving oxygen, if needed, will cure many of these problems.

The importance of providing a thermoregulated environment for the newborn cannot be overemphasized. Newborns have over three times the skin surface area to mass that an average adult does and will rapidly lose and gain heat to radiation, convection, and conduction. Radiation is the most important heat-transfer mechanism in newborns, so it is important to monitor the temperature of the room's walls when creating a thermally supportive atmosphere for newborns. Initially, a radiant heater controlled by an abdominal thermostat or being held next to the mother's skin covered by a blanket are the two most successful means of warming a newborn. Most infants have normal or slightly below normal temperatures on arrival in the nursery, because heat loss is more

Table 4.2   Assessment of vital signs in the neonate

Objective: To observe that the infant is maintaining vital signs that are compatible with an optimal transition to extrauterine life.

Policy:

1. Vital signs are taken every 30 min times 4. This procedure is to be initiated 30 min after delivery, even if still in the delivery room.
2. Vital signs are taken on all infants once per 8-hr shift (axillary temperature, heart rate, respirations) until discharge from term nursery.
3. Temperature and respirations are taken when an infant is scored with the neonatal abstinence syndrome (NAS) protocol. Infants on NAS scoring who are started on neonatal opium are to be placed on either an apnea monitor or a cardiorespiratory monitor until discharged from the nursery.
4. A temperature is taken every 3 hr, before each feeding, for any infant receiving phototherapy.
5. Infants receiving IV antibiotics should have vital signs (axillary temp, heart rate, respirations) taken at least every 4 hr until antibiotic therapy has been discontinued. Once antibiotic therapy has been discontinued, infant will have vital signs obtained once per shift unless physician orders more frequent vital signs.
6. All infants born to mothers who are GBS positive and inadequately treated or GBS unknown should have vitals signs taken (temperature, heart rate, respirations) every 4 hr until the laboratory results of the CBC/differential and CRP are back and physician has been notified.
7. Additional vital signs are taken when they have been ordered by the physician and for any infant who demonstrates signs/symptoms of illness, distress, or temperature instability.

common than heat gain. Persistently abnormal body temperature can lead to lethargy, irritability, seizures, brain damage, and even death.

Once the infant has been at a stable temperature for 2 hours, he or she can be bathed and, after a further short period of monitoring, dressed, wrapped, and placed in an open bassinet. Any infant that cannot maintain his or her own temperature and any febrile infant (temperature greater than 100.0°F rectally) requires immediate clinical and laboratory evaluation, because temperature instability and fever may be early indicators of sepsis.

Hydration is rarely a problem in newborns, because when they are born they are greater than 90% water by weight. In fact, the newborn normally has a diuresis immediately after birth, which causes a weight loss of 3% to 10% during the first 72 hours of life. Unfortunately, if the child has other problems that may cause high-output cardiac failure,

Table 4.3   Obtaining a temperature

Steps in Procedure	Points to be Emphasized
Axillary Temperature • Cover electronic thermometer probe with plastic cover and hold firmly against axilla with arm pressed against side. • Axillary temperatures are routinely done. • Normal newborn axillary temperatures should range between 97.7°F and 99.4°F. • If temperature is below 97°F, place infant under radiant warmer or in isolette. Notify physician of persistent low temperature.	• Wear gloves when caring for unwashed newborn. • Rectal temperatures may be warranted to validate fever or hypothermia.
Rectal Temperature • Obtain electronic thermometer. Use the red top probe for obtaining rectal temperatures. Put on unsterile gloves and remove infant's diaper. • Stabilize infant by grasping ankles and folding knees gently back onto abdomen. • Lubricate the end of the covered probe with water-soluble lubricant. Place approximately 1/2 in. of the lubricated probe gently into the infant's rectum and hold in place until the thermometer displays a reading.	• Make sure to place a new plastic cover over the thermometer probe prior to taking infant's temperature. • A rectal temperature of 100.4°F is considered the equivalent of an axillary temperature of 99.4°F and is considered a fever.

such as an artereovenous malformation (AVM), high-output congenital heart disease, or severe anemia (following a severe intrauterine hemolysis), the high-fluid state of the newborn may lead to irreversible congestive heart failure. Primary signs of congestive heart failure are persistent tachycardia and dependent edema. Treatment with diuretics after consultation with a pediatric cardiologist may alleviate the problem long enough to permit transfer to a high-risk facility. Dehydration because of poor feeding is discussed in Chapter 26.

Table 4.4   Measuring pulse and respiratory rate

Apical pulse
- Using appropriately sized stethoscope, count apical pulse for one full min.
- Observe for regularity, rhythm, and presence of extra sounds.

- In the neonate, tachycardia is defined as a resting heart rate >160 beats per min (bpm). Bradycardia is defined as a resting heart rate ≤110 bpm within the first 24 hr of life. After 24 hr of life, neonatal heart rates may temporarily dip down to 100 bpm, especially during sleep.
- Point of maximum intensity is located lateral to left nipple at third or fourth interspace at the midclavicular line.

Respiratory rate
- Observe rise and fall of abdomen. Count respiratory rate for one full min.

- Normal respiratory rate in the neonate is 20–60 breaths per min. Tachypnea is a resting rate >60 breaths per min.

Documentation
- Chart vital signs on newborn record. Document in notes alterations from normal, interventions, and response.

- Observe that rise and fall of chest is synchronous. Seesaw movements and retractions warrant physician notification.

SUGGESTED READING

Fletcher, MA. *Physical diagnosis in neonatology.* Philadelphia: Lippincott, 1997.

CHAPTER 5
Common Malformations Affecting Transition
Mae M. Coleman

When newborn resuscitation is failing, think about physical obstructions to airflow.

Some newborn malformations require immediate stabilization in the delivery room. Proper treatment greatly improves their outcome. Five specific malformations are listed in Table 5.1.

Choanal atresia is a rare congenital blockage of one or both of the posterior nares by a membrane of bone or cartilage. Newborn babies are obligate nasal breathers. They do not know to open their mouths to breathe if the nares are blocked. Infants with bilateral choanal atresia present with severe respiratory distress in the first few minutes of life. If both nares are obstructed, the infant must be stabilized immediately by securing an airway. This is done by either intubating the infant with an endotracheal tube or inserting a properly fitting oral or nasopharyngeal airway. See Table 5.2.

Infants with the *Pierre-Robin syndrome* have an abnormally small jaw, which forces the tongue against the posterior pharynx, in turn causing airway obstruction. The infant must be stabilized either by intubation with an endotracheal tube or by insertion of an oral airway.

Congenital diaphragmatic hernia is a serious malformation in which the abdominal viscera are displaced into the thoracic cavity through a defect in the diaphragm. The lung on the same side as the herniation develops abnormally and to small size. The infant with this anomaly will have respiratory distress, decreased breath sounds on the affected side, and a scaphoid-appearing abdomen due to displacement of the abdominal organs. The infant suspected of congenital diaphragmatic hernia should not be given bag-mask ventilation through the mouth. He or she should be intubated as soon as possible and have a nasogastric

Table 5.1	Common malformations

- Choanal atresia
- Pierre-Robin syndrome (or any other syndrome with small mandible)
- Congenital diaphragmatic hernia
- Abdominal wall defects
    - Omphalocele
    - Gastroschisis
- Neural tube defects

Table 5.2   Airway sizes

Type of Airway	Choosing Size
Oral	Flange at front of teeth, tip should reach until angle of jaw
Nasopharygeal	Diameter: 24 or 36 F
	Length: Tip of nose to angle of jaw
Endotreacheal tube	Diameter: <5 lb, 2.5 or 3.0 F; ≥5 lb, 3.0 or 3.5 F
	Length: 2.5 diameter tube, 7–8 cm; 3.0 diameter tube, 8.5–9.5 cm; 3.5 diameter tube, 10–11 cm

tube placed. It is best to transport these infants to the neonatal intensive care unit without delay. If it is known prior to delivery that a congenital diaphragmatic hernia exists, then the mother should be transferred to a tertiary care hospital, if possible, prior to the baby's delivery.

The two *abdominal wall defects* requiring stabilization in the delivery room are omphalocele and gastroschisis. These result from failure of fusion of the abdominal wall folds during embryonic development. The omphalocele is contained in a covering sac, with the umbilical cord inserted onto the central portion. The gastroschisis is usually a smaller defect without a covering sac and found lateral to a normally attached umbilicus. Either defect, when present at birth, should be covered by sterile gauze soaked in sterile normal saline. A sterile bag should be placed on the infant from the bottom of the feet to just above the abdominal wall defect and fastened. This maneuver prevents contamination and helps to control infection.

The most common *neural tube defect* is spina bifida cystica, also known as a meningomyelocele. This is a herniation of a sac containing cerebrospinal fluid, meninges, spinal cord, and other neural elements through abnormally fused vertebrae. The defect can occur at any position down the length of the spine. The defect must be covered with sterile gauze soaked in sterile normal saline. The infant must then be placed in a sterile bag, fastened above the defect to prevent contamination and help control infection. Because of the high incidence of development of latex allergy in these patients, latex-free gloves and equipment should routinely be used when handling these patients.

SUGGESTED READING

Fanaroff AA, Martin RJ. *Neonatal-perinatal medicine: diseases of the fetus and infant,* 6th ed. St. Louis, MO: Mosby, 1997.

Schwartz MW, ed. *Clinical handbook of pediatrics,* 2nd ed. Baltimore: Williams & Wilkins, 1999.

Botto LD, Moore CA, Khoury MJ, Erickson JD. Neural-tube defects. *New Engl J Med* 1999;341:1509–1519.

CHAPTER 6

Tachypnea and Respiratory Distress

Mae M. Coleman

*The most common presenting symptom
of illness in the well nursery
is respiratory distress.*

Respiratory distress in the newborn can be a symptom of disturbance in any of the major organ systems. Although there is no single algorithm for the evaluation of the newborn exhibiting respiratory distress, the pathways of Fig. 6.1 and Table 6.1 present a basic approach. The information in Table 6.2 will help illustrate the magnitude of this common problem.

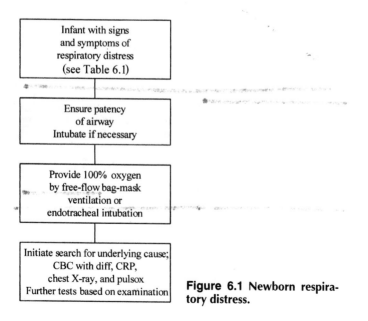

Figure 6.1 Newborn respiratory distress.

Table 6.1   Signs and symptoms of respiratory distress in the newborn

- Tachypnea (respirations >60 per min)
- Retractions
- Nasal flaring
- Grunting
- Poor inspiration
- Decreased oxygen saturation
- Central cyanosis
- Apnea

Table 6.2   Differential diagnosis of respiratory distress in the newborn

System	Diseases

Pulmonary	• Respiratory distress syndrome (RDS; hyaline membrane disease)
	• Transient tachypnea of the newborn (TTN)
	• Pneumonia
	• Chemical pneumonitis
	    Meconium aspiration
	    Amniotic fluid aspiration
	• Pneumothorax
	• Pleural effusion
	• Congenital malformations
	    Lobar emphysema
	    Cystic adenomatoid malformation
	    Lung sequestration
	• Diaphragmatic hernia

Airway	• Laryngomalacia • Choanal atresia • Pierre-Robin syndrome • Micrognathia • Tracheoesophageal fistula • Vascular ring
Cardiovascular	• Cyanotic and congenital heart disease • Congestive heart failure (CHF) • Arteriovenous malformation (AVM) • Persistent fetal circulation (pulmonary hypertension of the newborn)

(continued)

Table 6.2   (*Continued*)

System	Diseases
Neurologic	• Meningitis • Hypoxic-ischemic encephalopathy (HIE) • Intracranial hemorrhage • Hydrocephalus • Neuromuscular disease • Central hypoventilation • Apnea of prematurity
Hematologic	• Anemia • Polycythemia
Infectious	• Bacteremia • Viremia

Miscellaneous	• Hypothermia
	• Hypoglycemia
	• Maternal medications
	    Narcotics
	    Anesthesia
	    Hypermagnesemia
	• Acid–base imbalance
	• Electrolyte disturbances

SUGGESTED READING

Fanaroff AA, Martin RJ. *Neonatal-perinatal medicine: diseases of the fetus and infant,* 6th ed. St. Louis, MO: Mosby, 1997.

Schwartz MW, ed. *Clinical handbook of pediatrics,* 2nd ed. Baltimore: Williams & Wilkins, 1999.

CHAPTER 7

Hypoglycemia in the Delivery Room

Gary A. Emmett

> *WNL can mean either Within Normal Limits or We Never Looked. In newborns, forgetting to check serum glucose levels can lead to disaster.*

Hypoglycemia (low blood glucose level) may occur in any newborn. The primary problem may be lack of glucose stores, hyperinsulinemia, or both. Treatment pathways are presented in Fig. 7.1. As seen in Table 7.1, infants who received inadequate nutrition in utero will have a lack of glycogen stores that can be used to support the serum glucose level, whereas infants exposed to high maternal glucose levels will have high levels of insulin suppressing the serum glucose level.

Prolonged low serum glucose levels after birth may result in neurological damage. This association has prompted extensive research into the treatment of neonatal hypoglycemia. Management of neonatal hypoglycemia starts with the identification of those newborns at risk, performing glucose level determinations, and initiating therapy. Although the blood glucose concentration at which the brain is permanently affected is unknown, it is generally accepted that levels less than 40 to 45 mg/dL are abnormal. If quick methods show hypoglycemia, laboratory confirmation is necessary.

The definition of hypoglycemia may differ according to gestational age and degree of illness of the infant. Glucose levels should be determined during the first 1 to 3 hours after birth in high-risk infants and infants with symptoms such as jitteriness, high-pitched cry, and clonus. See Table 7.2 for a complete list of symptoms.

Newborns exposed to high glucose levels in utero, essentially infants of diabetic mothers, develop hyperinsulinemia. These infants become ill more quickly with hypoglycemia and are less likely to respond to oral glucose. Most of these newborns are very large, but if the mother has poor blood flow to the placenta, one may find an average sized or small baby with excess insulin.

If a glucose level is found to be less than 40 to 45, the child should be given oral formula ad lib. Glucose should be rechecked 15 minutes after the feeding and again 1 or 2 hours later if symptoms persist. In an infant where hyperinsulinemia is suspected, oral glucose is usually insufficient to prevent recurrence of symptoms, and an intravenous line with 10% dextrose solution (D10W), 5 to 10 mL/kg initially, followed by a continuous infusion of glucose at 4 to 10 mg/kg/minute. Glucagon (0.02 mg/kg IM or IV) may be given, but is often ineffective because of the limited hepatic glucose stores of newborns.

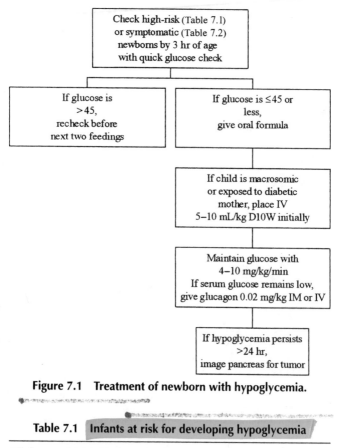

Figure 7.1   Treatment of newborn with hypoglycemia.

Table 7.1   Infants at risk for developing hypoglycemia

- Infants weighing less than 2,500 gm or greater than 4,000 gm at birth
- Infants less than 37 weeks or greater than 42 weeks of gestational age
- Infants of diabetic mothers
- Small for gestational age infants (SGA)
- Infants with neonatal problems such as respiratory distress, hypothermia, hypoxia
- Infants of mothers taking tocolytic agents, steroids, oral antidiabetic agents, illicit drugs
- Poor transition
- Maternal untreated endocrine and metabolic disorders
- Infants with chromosome disorders

Table 7.2   Symptoms of hypoglycemia

If any of the following signs or symptoms are noted, a blood glucose level should be determined and the practitioner notified:

- Tremors, jitteriness, irritability
- Hypertonia, hypotonia
- High-pitched, weak cry
- Eye rolling, staring, or other signs of seizure activity
- Lethargy and/or poor feeding
- Cyanosis/apneic spells
- Pallor, hypothermia
- Cardiomegaly, cardiac failure
- Difficulties with waking

If the child is still hypoglycemic, one must think about unusual causes of neonatal hypoglycemia, such as focal adenomatous hyperplasia of pancreatic β cells or other tumors of the pancreas. Congenital hypopituitarism can present with hypoglycemia and microphallus. Beckwith-Wiedemann syndrome (see Chapter 22) with its triad of macrosomia, abdominal wall defects, and macroglossia presents 50% of the time with intractable hypoglycemia.

If IV glucose fails to resolve the hypoglycemia, intractable disease may have to be treated with diazoxide and/or octreotide, which inhibit the action potential of the pancreatic β cell. In extreme cases, subtotal pancreotectomy may be required.

SUGGESTED READINGS

Schwartz MW, ed. *The 5-minute pediatric consult,* 2nd ed. Philadelphia: Lippincott, 2000:450–451.

Part II

Infectious Disease

CHAPTER 8
Tuberculosis
Gary A. Emmett

To people in the United States, tuberculosis is a disease of the 19th century, but its prevalence in much of the world makes it very much a 21st century problem.

Asymptomatic mothers who during pregnancy have a positive purified protein deriative (tuberculin; PPD), normal chest X-ray, and history of contact with a contagious person should receive isoniazid for 9 months. The therapy should not begin until after the end of the first trimester of the pregnancy. Pyridoxine (vitamin B_6) must be given to all pregnant women on isoniazid to prevent congenital spinal cord defects in their children. Isoniazid, ethambutol, and rifampin are considered safe for the fetus. If the mother has active tuberculosis, these should be used. On the other hand, streptomycin should not be used during pregnancy because of ototoxic effects on the fetus.

Pregnant women who have only pulmonary manifestations of tuberculosis are not likely to affect their infant in utero, but can easily infect the child after birth. If the mother has extrapulmonary tuberculosis, the child may have disseminated tuberculosis, although this outcome is exceedingly rare. If a child is suspected of having congenital tuberculosis, the workup in Table 8.1 should be followed, and the child should be treated promptly. No matter what the outcome of the newborn's PPD, if the mother has active extrapulmonary TB, then the child should be treated with isoniazid, rifampin, pyrazinamide, and an aminoglycoside.

The newborn's practitioner should inquire about tuberculosis if any of the criteria in Table 8.2 are positive. If tuberculosis or suspected tuberculosis is present in the home, *The Red Book*, 26th edition, suggests the treatment algorithm in Table 8.3. Consult the local public health authorities for details whenever treating active tuberculosis in the United States.

After the child is on isoniazid for 3 or 4 months and congenital tuberculosis is excluded, repeat the PPD. If the PPD is negative, finish 9 months of just isoniazid. If the PPD is positive, then the complete infant TB workup must be repeated. During active tuberculosis treatment, the child should be reassessed at least monthly.

Table 8.1 Workup of suspected congenital disseminated tuberculosis

- PPD
- Chest X-ray
- Lumbar puncture
- Tuberculosis cultures of cerebrospinal fluid (CSF), blood, and trachea
- Histological examination/culture of placenta for M tuberculosis
- HIV testing for mother and child
- Complete maternal tuberculosis workup

Treatment

- After birth, all the tuberculosis medications may be used, including streptomycin. Regime depends on sensitivities of culture (mother or child), but it always includes isoniazid.
- If CSF cultures are positive, corticocosteroids should be added to anti-TB regime.

Table 8.2 Infants with an increased risk of acquiring tuberculosis

- History of positive PPD in household
- Mother was born, or a member of her household was born, in high tuberculosis prevalent areas of the world (Africa, South and East Asia, Central and South America, Native American areas, the Pacific Islands)
- Mother or member of her household has:
  HIV infection
  Homelessness
  Used street drugs
  Been incarcerated or institutionalized
  Been migrant farm workers
  Traveled to high prevalence areas of the world listed above

Table 8.3   Level of TB exposure at home and infant workup/treatment

Level of Home Exposure	Workup/Treatment of Infant
● Mother/household contact has (+) PPD, normal CXR	Everyone in household should have PPDs and CXR done. Child may be discharged home.
● Mother/household contact has (+) PPD, abnormal CXR consistent with TB	Infant should be completely separated from individual who has (+) CXR until person has been treated for 2 full weeks.
● Mother/household contact has (+) PPD, abnormal CXR not consistent with TB, and is not thought to have active TB after full workup	Treat the (+) individual, follow infant and all others in household over time, but no separation necessary.
● Mother/household contact has (+) PPD, abnormal CXR, and clinical and/or radiographic evidence of contagious TB	A public health emergency. Full workup of everyone in home. Evaluate infant as in Table 8.1. Treat (+) individual and infant. Infant may remain in house if taking isoniazid. If multiresistant TB is suspected, infant must be separated from home, and consider giving infant BCG immunization.

SUGGESTED READING

Pickering LK, ed. *The red book,* 26th ed. Chicago: American Academy of Pediatrics, 2003.

CHAPTER 9
Prevention of Group B Streptococcal Disease

Judith A. Turow

In the 3-year gestation of this book, this chapter has been revised more times than any other chapter, because the "best practice" in this area is still somewhat hazy. Dr. Turow has made a serious attempt to synthesize a consistent whole from the conflicting advice available.

Since the 1970s, group B streptococcus (GBS) has been one of the leading causes of illness and death among newborns. In 1992, the American Academy of Pediatrics (AAP) developed a guideline for GBS that was poorly received and often ignored. In an attempt to have consensus, the AAP, American College of Obstetrics and Gynecology (ACOG), and US Centers for Disease Control and Prevention (CDC) created guidelines in 1996–1997 that produced a more unified approach to the pregnant women with GBS and the newborn of such a mother. To answer questions raised since the last writing, in 2002, the CDC again updated these guidelines. This chapter clarifies the CDC's approach to a mother who is either GBS-positive or GBS-unknown at the time of delivery.

The antibiotic treatment of GBS-positive mothers has resulted in a marked decrease in early onset GBS sepsis over the last decade in the United States. GBS is a gram-positive organism that causes beta-hemolysis on sheep agar. I (Ia, Ib/c), II, and III are the important types in neonatal sepsis. Newborn group B streptococcal disease (GBSD) is divided into early-onset group B streptococcal disease (EOGBSD) and late-onset group B streptococcal disease (LOGBSD). EOGBSD occurs in the first week of life, and LOGBSD occurs in the second week through approximately the third month of life. *Intrapartum treatment of mothers has been proven to protect against EOGBSD, but not against LOGBSD.*

This chapter discusses the prevention and detection of EOGBSD only. Additional guidelines and details for the treatment of the mothers in both premature and full-term labor can be found in the CDC guidelines in this chapter's suggested reading.

The current CDC recommendations suggest testing *all* mothers for GBS in the 35th to 37th week of gestation. Additionally, current CDC recommendations suggest treating mothers during labor (intrapartum prophylaxis or IAP) if they have:

Table 9.1   Intrapartum prophylaxis indications

Intrapartum prophylaxis is indicated for:

1. Previous infant with invasive GBS disease
2. GBS bacteriuria during current pregnancy
3. Positive GBS screening culture during current pregnancy (unless a planned Caesarean section delivery in the absence of labor or amniotic membrane rupture is performed)
4. Unknown GBS status (culture not done, incomplete, or results unknown) and any of the following:
   a. Delivery at <37 wk gestation
   b. Amniotic membrane rupture ≥18 hr
   c. Intrapartum temperature ≥100.4°F (≥38.0°C)

Intrapartum prophylaxis is not indicated for:

5. Previous pregnancy with a positive GBS screening culture (unless a culture was also positive during the current pregnancy)
6. Planned Caesarean delivery performed in the absence of labor or membrane rupture (regardless of the maternal GBS culture status)
7. Negative vaginal and rectal GBS screening culture in late gestation during the current pregnancy, regardless of intrapartum risk factors

If intrapartum prophylaxis is indicated, and is not given, or duration is <4 hr, obtain a full diagnostic evaluation and start empiric treatment.

1. Positive GBS screening culture during current pregnancy (Screening for GBS is not required if a Caesarean section delivery without labor or amniotic rupture is planned.)

2. GBS bacteriuria during this pregnancy

3. History of a previous infant with invasive GBS disease

4. Unknown GBS screening culture (a culture was not done, is incomplete, or its results are unknown) and any of the following risk factors:
   a. Delivery at <37 weeks' gestation
   b. Amniotic membrane rupture at 18 hours
   c. Intrapartum temperature of 100.4°F (38.0°C)

The 2002 CDC report recommends that it is *not* necessary to treat mothers in full-term labor if the baby has the following lack of risk factors:

1. Previous pregnancy with a positive GBS screening culture (unless a new culture was positive during a current pregnancy)

Table 9.2 Adequate dose of intrapartum antibiotics to prevent GBS disease

Antibiotic prophylaxis:
Penicillin G, 5 million units IV initial dose, then 2.5 million units IV every 4 hr until delivery, or

Alternative
Ampicillin, 2 g IV initial dose, then 1 g IV every 4 hr until delivery
If penicillin allergic[+] (in patients not at high risk for anaphylaxis), administer Cefazolin,[++] 2 g IV initial dose, then 1 g IV every 8 hr until delivery

Patients at high risk for anaphylaxis:
(GBS susceptible to clindamycin and erythromycin [+++])
Clindamycin, 900 mg IV (preferred) every 8 hr until delivery
or
Erythromycin, 500 mg IV every 6 hr until delivery
(GBS resistant to clindamycin or erythromycin, or susceptibility unknown)
Vancomycin[++] 1 g IV every 12 hr until delivery

[+]Penicillin allergy should be assessed to determine whether a high risk for anaphylaxis is present. Penicillin-allergic patients at high risk for anaphylaxis are those who have experienced immediate hypersensitiviy to penicillin including a history of penicillin-related anaphylaxis; other high-risk patients are those with asthma or other diseases that would make anaphylaxis more dangerous to treat, such as those patients being treated with beta-adrenergic-blocking drugs.

[++]Cefazolin is preferred over vancomycin for women with a history of penicillin allergy other than immediated hypersensitiviy reactions, and pharmacologic data suggest it acheives effective intramniotic concentrations. Vancomycin should be reserved fo penicillin-allergic women at high risk for anaphylaxis.

[+++]If laboratory facilites are adequate, test for clindamycin and erythromycin susceptibility; resistance to erythromycin is often, but not always, associated with clindamycin resistance. If a strain is resistant to erythromycin but appears susceptible to clindamycin, it may still have inducible resistance to clindamycin. (From prevention of group B beta-hemolytic sepsis. *MMWR* 2002 Aug 16:10.)

2. Planned Caesarian delivery performed in the absence of labor or membrane rupture (regardless of the maternal GBS culture status)

3. Negative vaginal and rectal GBS screening culture in late gestation during the current pregnancy, regardless of intrapartum risk factors

If intrapartum prophylaxis is indicated (Table 9.1) and is not given, or the duration is considered inadequate, the recommendation is to treat the baby as indicated in Fig 9.1. See Table 9.2 for adequate doses and durations for intrapartum antibiotics to prevent GBS disease.

In the protocol used at the Thomas Jefferson University Hospital (TJUH) newborn nursery, when intrapartum prophylaxis of the GBS-positive mother is indicated for prevention of GBSD, then two additional questions must be asked: "Was the mother treated for suspected or actual chorioamnionitis?" and "Does the infant appear ill?" If the answer to either question is yes, a full septic workup is warranted. The full evaluation includes a complete blood count with differential (CBC), a C-reactive program (CRP), a blood culture, a chest X-ray (if the child is in respiratory distress), and, at the discretion of the examiner, a lumbar puncture.

If the infant appears well, the practitioner asks, "Is the newborn under or over 35 weeks?" If the newborn is less than 35 weeks, the practitioner performs a limited evaluation: a CBC, a CRP, and a blood culture. The infant should be treated with antibiotics, such as ampicillin (100 mg/kg/12 hours) and gentamycin (4 mg/kg/24 hours) until the blood culture is negative for at least 48 hours. Table 9.3 lists the recommended empiric treatment for newborns exposed to GBS.

If the child is 35 weeks or greater, the practitioner determines if the maternal intrapartum treatment is adequate (used penicillin, ampicillin, or cefazolin starting more than 4 hours prior to birth). If maternal treatment is inadequate, one performs the same limited evaluation as for the untreated child.

Table 9.3	Recommended empiric treatment for newborns exposed to GBS

Ampicillin, plus aminoglycoside.
Ampicillin 100 mg/kg/dose, given every 12 hr. Total daily dose is 200 mg/kg/day.
Gentamycin dosed for age;

$\leq$29 weeks	5 mg/kg/day	every 48 hr
30–33 weeks	4.5 mg/kg/day	every 48 hr
34–37 weeks	4 mg/kg/day	every 36 hr
$\geq$38 weeks	4 mg/kg/day	every 24 hr
Trough level from the 3rd dose	(trough 0.5–1 mcg/mL)	
Peak level	(peak 5–12 mcg/mL, or C_{max}/MIC ratio greater than 8:1)	

Duration of therapy depends on extent of disease:
   If baby is asymptomatic and culture(s) are negative, treat patient for 2–3 days.
   If symptomatic and there are maternal risk factors, treat patient for a 7–10 days.
   If blood culture is positive, treat patient for 7–10 days.
   If CSF culture is positive, treat patient for 21 days.

Treatment of Children Whose Mother is GBS (+)

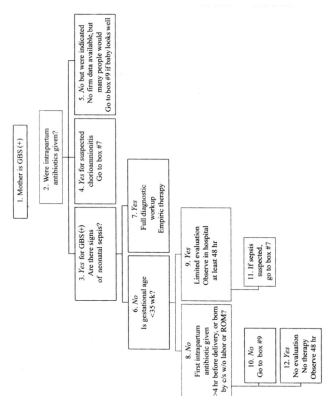

1. Mother is GBS (+)

2. Were intrapartum antibiotics given?

3. *Yes* for GBS(+)
Are there signs of neonatal sepsis?

4. *Yes* for suspected chorioamnionitis
Go to box #7

5. *No* but were indicated
No firm data available, but many people would Go to box #9 if baby looks well

6. *No*
Is gestational age <35 wk?

7. *Yes*
Full diagnostic workup
Empiric therapy

8. *No*
First intrapartum antibiotic given >4 hr before delivery, or born by c/s w/o labor or ROM?

9. *Yes*
Limited evaluation
Observe in hospital at least 48 hr

10. *No*
Go to box #9

11. If sepsis suspected, go to box #7

12. *Yes*
No evaluation
No therapy
Observe 48 hr

Options for maternal antibiotics include penicillin, ampicillin, cefazolin, vancomycin, clindamycin, or erythromycin. Only penicillin and ampicillin strategies for prophylaxis have been clinically tested. GBS resistance for those two drugs has not yet been shown. Similarly, the minimal inhibitory concentrations (MICs) of invasive GBS isolates for cefazolin have been low in 1996–2002, suggesting that GBS is currently also susceptible to this drug. Conversely, there has been increasing resistance shown among GBS isolates for erythromycin and clindamycin. Vancomycin resistance for GBS has not been shown; however, the CDC does not believe that there is sufficient evidence of its efficacy to ensure its adequate treatment of GBS. Hence in the new guidelines, only penicillin, ampicillin, and cefazolin are listed as appropriate intrapartum antibiotics, and even these must be given to the mother starting at least 4 hours prior to birth.

New to the 2002 guidelines are provisions for discharging an infant earlier than the standard 48 hours of life. If the infant is healthy appearing and at least 38 weeks gestation, the caregiver has been taught to recognize sepsis, and the mother was given adequate treatment with appropriate antibiotics, the infant may be discharged home after 24 hours of life. The caveat is that a caretaker who is fully instructed in signs and symptoms of an infant's distress will be at home to observe the child, and that all the other discharge criteria are met. If there is any question about these conditions, babies born to GBS-positive mothers

---

Figure 9.1
- If maternal GBS status is unknown, and risk factors are present, start in box #9 (delivery <37 weeks, ROM >18 hr, maternal temperature >100.4°F)
  - *Full diagnosis evaluation* includes:
  - CBC with differential
  - CRP
  - Blood culture
  - Chest X-ray if in respiratory distress
  - Spinal tap if sepsis is suspected
- *Limited diagnostic evaluation* has no chest X-ray or spinal tap
- Empiric therapy duration can be as short as 48 hours if blood work is negative, or as long as 10 days if a positive blood culture is obtained.
- Only penicillin, ampicillin, or cefazolin are recommended. If other antibiotics are given, do a limited evaluation as above, unless the specific maternal cultures have been proven sensitive to clindamycin, erythromycin, or vancomycin in prenatal testing.
- Healthy GBS (+) babies, >38 wk gestation, who received recommended intrapartum antibiotics >4 hr before delivery and are otherwise well may go home after 24 hr.

must be observed for 48 hours in the hospital. Also included are clearer provisions for treatment of children of mothers who have undergone Cesarean sections or whose GBS status is unknown.

For GBS unknown, the mother is treated for the risk factors listed. If the mother is undergoing a Caesarean section and has had active labor, or has had a prior rupture of membranes (ROM), she is treated by the protocol as her situation warrants (either GBS positive or GBS unknown, with or without risk factors).

Unless the baby is visibly ill, a diagnostic evaluation is usually done between 8 and 12 hours of age. If the results are questionable or mildly abnormal, they are repeated about every 12 hours, up to three times total.

Depending on the hospital, the CRP may be used in the limited evaluation. Although this is above and beyond the CDC guidelines, the CRP as a single test has a predictive value for EOGBSD of up to 97%, depending on the timing of the study and whether one performs it only once or in a series of three, every 12 to 24 hours. A single CRP at 8 to 24 hours of life has a sensitivity of almost 79% and a negative predictive value of 99%. For this reason, a CRP is used along with the limited evaluation in the first 8 to 12 hours of life.

At TJUH, if the CRP is greater than 3.0 and/or the white blood cell count shows an increased number of immature cells [bands/(bands + neutrophils) ratio > 0.2], we assess the child for signs and symptoms of sepsis, repeat the laboratory examinations immediately, and talk to the neonatologist. If the child is symptomatic at any time, the patient is transferred to the intensive care nursery. If the child has a CRP slightly greater than 3.0, and/or an I/T ratio that is elevated but less than 0.2, the practitioner should repeat the laboratory examinations. The practitioner should keep a close watch on the patient with repeat exams and frequent vital signs. If the practitioner remains unsure about the baby, the laboratory test may be repeated every 12 hours.

Black Box Warning!

Only adequately dosed penicillin, ampicillin, or cefazolin started at least 4 hours prior to delivery is considered fully effective in prevention of early-onset group B streptococcus disease. If any other antibiotic is used, or if these antibiotics are not started soon enough, consider doing a limited evaluation as described in Fig. 9.1

SUGGESTED READING

Prevention of group B beta-hemolytic sepsis. *MMWR* 2002 Aug 16.

C H A P T E R 10
Congenital Syphilis
Gary A. Emmett

Syphilis during pregnancy has a transmission rate approaching 100%.

Active congenital syphilis can cause death, prematurity, or even hydrops at birth, or it can present as late as age two years with the primary manifestations of skin lesions, snuffles, organomegaly, lymphadenopathy, and/or blood dyscrasias. Congenital syphilis can also cause pseudoparalysis, generalized edema, bone lesions, or peculiar skin ulcers.

Even if one never has the primary manifestations just noted, an untreated child with congenital syphilis can develop the late symptoms of syphilis, discussed later, up to 40 years after birth.

Syphilis is, thankfully, increasingly rare, but it is still maims untreated newborns. Because of its rare occurrence, practitioners are uncomfortable dealing with this disease. Following the pathway of Fig. 10.1 should minimize this discomfort. There are alternative treatment regimes, and in this instance, the *Red Book 2003* gives several treatment courses, but the regime in Fig. 10.1 is relatively straightforward, and, although it may be overtreating, it is safe.

All mothers must have a nontreponemal test result for syphilis (VDRL and RPR are the most commonly used) reported prior to discharge. If the RPR or VDRL is negative, then no further workup is performed on either mother or child.

If the nontreponemal test is positive, a treponemal test such as a FTA or a MHA must be done. If the treponemal test is negative, then the mother probably has a false-positive RPR, and a workup may be done for an antiself disease such as lupus or an alternative sphirocete such as the Lyme vector.

If both nontreponemal and treponemal tests are positive, then the mother has had syphilis or currently has syphilis. All children in this instance should have a thorough physical examination for signs of syphilis and a venous RPR or VDRL. Further workup (a lumbar puncture for cerebral spinal fluid including VDRL, a dark-field examination, protein, and cell count; long-bone radiographs; and CBC with platelet count) is indicated if the mother has any of the conditions cited in Table 10.1.

If the mother was not adequately treated (there was an insufficient dosage, she used an ineffective antibiotic, there is no documentation of treatment, or she was reinfected since receiving treatment), then treat the infant with parenteral aqueous penicillin G. Treatment is 50,000 units per kilogram per dose every 12 hours for a child less than 7 days old and every 8 hours if the child is greater than 7 days old. Treatment course is 10 days. If any day's medication is missed, then treatment must be started over again for the full 10 days.

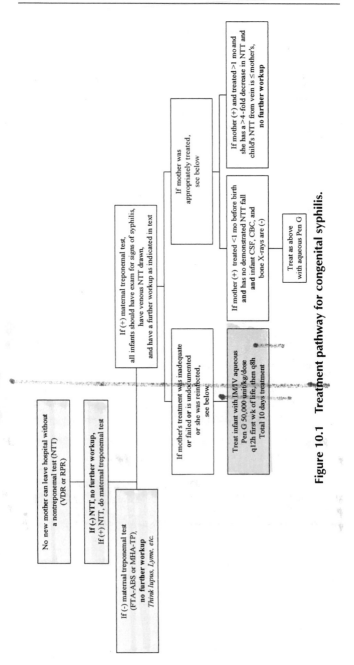

Figure 10.1 Treatment pathway for congenital syphilis.

Table 10.1   Maternal conditions indicating a full infant workup (CSF, CBC, platelets, long-bone films)

- Syphilis untreated, inadequately treated, or treatment undocumented
- Syphilis during pregnancy treated, but not with penicillin
- No fourfold fall in RPR or VDRL after seemingly adequate treatment
- Syphilis treated less than 1 mo prior to child's delivery
- Syphilis treated without documentation of follow-up
- Child's NTT test is fourfold greater than mother's
- Child has symptoms of syphilis

If the mother was appropriately treated more than 1 month prior to birth *and* she has a greater than fourfold decrease in the RPR or VDRL *and* the child's venous RPR or VDRL is less than or equal to the mother's, then no further workup or treatment is needed.

Maternal untreated syphilis during pregnancy is almost universally transmitted to the infant. This high degree of infectivity explains why no mother should ever leave the hospital without having her RPR or VDRL checked and why a newborn's practitioner should always choose to treat the child if the diagnosis is uncertain.

In acquired syphilis, the patient's disease is divided into three phases. *Primary syphilis* has chancres, which are painless papules that occur 2 weeks or more after exposure, primarily at the site of contact. These chancres turn into painless ulcers with significant regional adenitis. The chancre usually heals within 6 weeks. This phase is not seen in newborns.

Secondary syphilis results from a T. pallidum septicemia that occurs several weeks to 3 months after the primary chancres heal. The initial

Table 10.2   Early manifestations of congenital syphilis

Each of these symptoms occurs in 50% or less of patients
Listed from most common to least common
- Osteochondritis (may occur in any bone, leading most prominently to saddle nose and saber shins)
- Snuffles (chronic, profuse rhinitis)
- Rash (a desquamating rash most prominent on palms, soles, mouth, and anus—similar to the rashes seen in Kawasaki syndrome. Initially, epidermis at site of rash is teeming with spirochetes. Syphilis can have almost any rash.)
- Hepatosplenomegaly (with secondary anemia and jaundice)
- Neurologic abnormalities (Irritability primarily. After 3 mo of age, infected child has syphilitic meningitis 30% of time but may not display any neurologic symptoms even if meningitic.)

Table 10.3   Late manifestations of congenital syphilis

- Bone abnormalities—frontal bossing, saddle nose, prominent mandible with short maxilla, high arched palate, thick sternum, saber shins, and many others
- Teeth abnormalities—mulberry molars and Hutchinson incisors
- Interstitial keratitis (eye)
- Neurologic—eighth nerve deafness, tabes dorsalis, generalized weakness
- Gummas—granulomata of any tissue secondary to the pervasive end arteritis of late syphilis
- Aortic arteritis

symptoms (formally, early manifestations) in congenital syphilis are equivalent to this phase. These symptoms are listed in Table 10.2 and, most important, include T. pallidum meningitis up to 30% of the time. The multiple symptoms of secondary syphilis can come and go for 1 to 2 years.

Tertiary syphilis may present in protean manners, especially involving the nervous system, the heart, and the skin/soft tissue. The late manifestations of congenital syphilis (see Table 10.3) are equivalent to tertiary syphilis in acquired syphilis. Since many of these delayed symptoms are associated with hypersensitivity reactions of the patient and not with active infection, these symptoms are very difficult to treat and may not respond to antibiotics.

Although the vast majority of untreated children exposed to maternal syphilis will exhibit some early manifestations in the first 2 years of life, not all do. To make the diagnostic dilemma even more difficult, children can have no signs of syphilis for years after birth and still have the multiple late manifestations. The late manifestations of congenital syphilis can begin as late as adulthood. Eighth nerve deafness, as a first sign of congenital syphilis, has been reported as late as age 40. Most of the early manifestations are secondary to direct infection. Most of the late manifestations are secondary to endarteritis and/or autoimmune reactions of the host. The length of this abbreviated list demonstrates why this disease is called "the great imposter."

SUGGESTED READING

Azimi P. Spirochetal infections. *Nelson textbook of pediatrics,* 15th ed. Philadelphia: WB Saunders, 1996.

Pickering LK, ed. *The red book,* 26th ed. Chicago: American Academy of Pediatrics, 2003.

CDC treatment suggestions. <www.cdc.gov/nchstp/dstd/penicillinG .htm/>

C H A P T E R   11
The TORCH Syndrome
Gary A. Emmett

The TORCH syndrome is the best defined of the interuterine infections.

When a newborn is unstable or has difficulty going through transition, a practitioner should think about infection. Other than the obvious bacterial sepsis predominantly caused by group B streptococcus, E. coli, and L. monocytogenes, many viral causes of infection occur, and other less acute bacterial infections are possible. Five of these infections are grouped under the rubric TORCH syndrome as described in Table 11.1.

Certain physical findings are often found in these five diseases. Classic physical examination signs of these infections at birth are microcephaly, petechiae, and generalized small for gestational age. Any one of the findings in Table 11.2 would alert the practitioner to start a diagnostic work up for the TORCH diseases, but having two or more of these findings makes it much more likely that the search will have a positive outcome.

Toxoplasma gondii is an intracellular protozoan. This parasite lives in the cat but unfortunately can affect the central nervous system and other areas of a newborn. Congenital toxoplasmosis is usually a product of a mother's primary infestation during pregnancy. She has ingested the cysts of the parasite initially by the fecal (feline)/oral (human) route. In women who are severely immunocompromised, such as someone with HIV infection, the parasite can be communicated to the fetus in utero even if the mother has a chronic, not an acute, infection. The earlier in pregnancy that a mother has her primary infestation, the more severely infected the newborn will be. Pregnant women should avoid raw or almost raw meats and caring for cats if they are seronegative for toxoplasmosis. In areas of high incidence (France, for instance), prenatal toxoplasmosis titers are a must. About a third of newborns whose mother have a primary infestation during pregnancy will be affected.

The rate of congenital infection in the United States is less than one per one thousand births. The vast majority of affected children are asymptomatic at birth, but if untreated, more than 50% of these children will develop severe sequelae. Congenital effects include microcephaly, sensorineural hearing loss, retardation, seizures, and retinitis. Late effects include swollen glands, myocarditis, and meningitis. A newborn who has symptoms at birth is more likely to get the late sequelae than one who does not have congenital symptoms.

In congenital toxoplasmosis, physical examination finds microcephaly, chorioretinitis, hepatosplenomegaly, petechiae, and hearing loss. Physical findings of late manifestation include hepatosplenomegaly

Table 11.1 The TORCH syndrome

T	Toxoplasmosis
O	Others (primarily syphilis)
R	Rubella
C	Cytomegalic inclusion disease
H	Herpes

(a common finding in congenital infections), swollen glands, fever, and poor feeding. The definitive test is brain imaging showing intracerebral calcifications, but these can develop after birth, especially in disease acquired late in pregnancy. Also often present are thrombocytopenia, specific elevation of IgM or IgA for toxoplasmosis, elevated liver enzymes, and failure to pass vision or hearing screens.

Once toxoplasmosis is diagnosed, the therapeutic regime in Table 11.3 is suggested. This therapy must be given in all diagnosed patients for the first year of life. Folic acid is given to prevent anemia from the pyrimethamine and sulfadiazine, which are not innocuous in the newborn and must be monitored closely with frequent complete blood counts.

Other (syphilis) is treated in Chapter 10.

Rubella, German measles, is currently rare in the United States, because of the requirement for two measles shots prior to school entry. Because measles is easily available only in the combination vaccination for measles, mumps, and rubella (MMR), almost all students in the United States also receive two rubella vaccines before entering kindergarten. Because young children do not now get rubella, their mother and their mother's friends do not contract rubella during their pregnancies. Prior to mass vaccination, rubella was the leading cause of congenital deafness. In 1964–1965 in the United States, an epidemic resulted in over 20,000 confirmed cases of congenital rubella syndrome (CRS) and an estimated 2,100 stillbirths. In 2000, less than 200 cases of CRS occurred, primarily in Hispanic immigrants.

Table 11.2 Signs and symptoms of TORCH syndrome infections

- Microcephaly/macrocephaly (especially if inappropriate for family)
- IUGR (intrauterine growth retardation)
- Petechiae (thrombocytopenia)
- Abdominal organomegaly
- Retinitis
- Sensorineural hearing loss

Table 11.3   Treatment of toxoplasmosis-infected newborns

The optimal therapeutic regime has not been established in a controlled study
- Pyrimethamine:
     Loading—2 mg/kg/day for 2 days
     Maintenance—1 mg/kg/day for 12 mo
- Sulfadiazine: 100 mg/kg/day divided into two doses
- Folinic acid: 10 mg three times weekly (to prevent marrow suppression from the above medications)

Therapy is a full 12 months

It is usually assumed that people born after 1956 and who have no history of rubella immunization are susceptible to rubella until proven otherwise. All pregnant women should be tested for rubella titers, and those who are not immune should be reimmunized immediately after the birth of their baby. Because rubella is a live vaccine, it is not recommended during pregnancy, but there is no evidence that the rubella vaccine during pregnancy is a danger to the fetus.

Rubella itself is a mild disease. First, 2 to 3 weeks after exposure, the patient has adenitis behind the ears and on the back of the neck, mild fever, fatigue, and conjunctivitis. Second, 3 to 7 days later a maculopapular rash spreads down from the face and neck over the entire body and fades after several days. The patient is infectious 1 week prior and 1 week after the rash appears. In adolescents and adults, rubella sequelae include arthralgias, frank arthritis, and rarely, thrombocytopenia and encephalitis. The sequelae can also occur in adults with the rubella vaccine, but the onset of chronic arthritis has not been confirmed in these cases.

CRS occurs when mothers are infected in the first trimester of pregnancy, but sensorineural deafness may occur in isolation in later congenital infections. Children with the symptoms listed in Table 11.4 should be cultured for the virus. Because the patient may shed virus in

Table 11.4   Signs and symptoms of congenital rubella syndrome

- Sensorineural hearing loss
- Cataracts
- Retinopathy
- Patent ductus arteriosus

Occasionally
- Glaucoma
- Developmental delays
- Endocrinopathies

Table 11.5   Signs and symptoms of cytomegalic inclusion disease

- Intrauterine growth retardation (IUGR)
- Thrombocytopenia (plus occasional neutropenia)
- Hepatosplenomegaly (with jaundice and/or hepatitis)
- CNS abnormalities
    Sensorineural hearing loss
    Intracranial calcification
    Microcephaly
    Partial obstruction to ventricular fluid flow
- Chorioretinitis

secretions (nasal secretions, urine, spinal fluid) for a year, delayed diagnosis is possible. Culture, PCR, and rising IgG titers (after 6 months of life) are all good indicators of disease. There is no effective therapy for CRS, but diagnosis is important both to prevent spread of disease and to institute specific therapy for findings such as impaired hearing or vision.

Cytomegalovirus (CMV) is a ubiquitous DNA herpes virus that almost everyone will acquire at some time in life. In older children and adults, it causes a mononucleosislike syndrome of generalized adenopathy, prolonged intermittent fever, and chronic fatigue. It has been estimated that 1 in 100 babies is born with a positive urine for CMV but only 1 or 2000 or less has what is termed cytomegalic inclusion disease (CMID). This congenital infection (the symptoms of which are listed in Table 11.5) is very much like the other TORCH infections listed earlier, but because of CMID's widespread nature, it is currently the most common cause of congenital hearing loss. Even worse is that it may not be obvious at first that the child is affected (the child may even pass its hospital hearing test) and will still cause progressive deafness in the first 2 years of life.

A CMV-infected individual can secrete virus from all mucous membranes and urine for a year or more (and because this virus, like many herpes viruses, can exist in the nervous system for many years, it can also be secreted at various later times in life). But the most accurate diagnostic method for demonstrating CMID is a CMV culture of the infant's urine in the first 2 weeks of life, because after 2 weeks, the virus may be present from perinatally acquired CMV.

The treatment of CMID is described in Table 11.6. Remember that this treatment is virostatic and does not eliminate the virus from the body. Treatment is indicated in ill infants if immunocompromised to mitigate chorioretinitis, hepatitis, pneumonitis, and enteritis. No treatment is indicated for asymptomatic children with CMID, but may or may not be indicated after studies underway are completed.

Table 11.6   Treatment of cytomegalic inclusion disease in immunocompromised infants

Ganciclovir	5 mg/kg IV q12h × 2 wk follow in HIV with 30 mg/kg/dose PO TID

- Follow-up is with reduced doses until child is no longer immunocompromised.
- Ganciclovir is myelosuppressive, so follow CBCs weekly at first.
- If virus is resistant to ganciclovir or to myelosuppressive, foscarnet or cidofovir can be used. Consult a pediatric infectious disease specialist before therapy.

Herpes simplex genital exposure occurs in more than 10% of sexually active American women. Over 20% of adults are seropositive for herpes type II. This virus can be latent in peripheral nerves, as can all herpes viruses, for periods of months to years and suddenly reappear. Antivirals suppress, but do not eliminate, herpes infections. Herpes simplex type I is usually above the waist and type II below the waist, but both can be active in the vagina and cause problems in the newborn.

Congenital herpes has a moderate to poor outcome even if treated promptly. The outcome, if not treated promptly, is dire. Following Table 11.7, think of congenital herpes if vesicles are found, if the baby is lethargic, or if the baby has the common findings of the TORCH infections (microcephaly, chorioretinitis, organomegaly). Most important, if there is a history of vaginal herpes, and the child is irritable or not eating well or having trouble arousing, check the baby for herpes. A classic presentation is a child admitted for "rule out" sepsis who does not get better on antibiotics. Herpes can appear in the newborn as skin and eye lesions, as encephalitis, or as septicemia. Children usually become ill between 7 and 21 days, but systemic congenital herpes can appear as late as 6 weeks. PCR is the best diagnostic tool in the newborn, but herpes grows well in culture also. Once the diagnosis of congenital herpes is entertained, treatment should be started as soon as possible. See Table 11.8.

Acyclovir at 30 mg per kilogram per dose every 6 hours IV is the drug of choice for invasive congenital herpes infection. Trifluridine or

Table 11.7   Clues to the diagnosis of congenital herpes

- History of mother with vaginal herpes and any problems in the child
- Vesicles (especially on presenting parts)
- Microcephaly
- Hepatosplenomegaly
- Chorioretinitis

Table 11.8   Treatment of congenital herpes simplex

Acyclovir   30 mg/kg/dose q4–6h for 14–21 days

- If resistant to acyclovir, try foscarnet 40 mg/kg/dose q8h
- If retinitis, try trifluridine eye drops TID

other antiviral eye drops may be indicated. Early treatment increases survival rates from 50% to almost 75%. Unfortunately, serious CNS disability is still close to 25%, even in treated babies. Children with encephalitis have a much lower survival rate (about 30%).

How can we prevent this awful disease? By delivering babies born to known active vaginal herpes mothers by Caesarean section. Also by keeping babies with exposure away from other newborns. Strict isolation is not necessary, but close observation is.

SUGGESTED READING

Pickering LK, ed. *The red book,* 26th ed. Chicago: American Academy of Pediatrics, 2003.

Schwartz MW, ed. *The 5-minute pediatric consult.* Philadelphia: Lippincott, 2000.

Human Immunodeficiency Virus (HIV)

Sue Jue and Nicholas Slamon

In resource-rich parts of the world, we can now prevent congenital HIV in most children.

In the best of all possible worlds, all women of childbearing age would have prenatal HIV testing done, as in Fig. 12.1. Practitioners should encourage all mothers to be tested for HIV, but in most states, we cannot force them to do so. At the time of delivery, the mother's HIV status must be available, especially for those in high-risk groups. See Table 12.1.

If the mother is HIV positive, in an ideal world she would be treated prior to delivery. If the mother is HIV positive, the newborn should receive AZT prophylaxis in the first few hours of life and continue the therapy for 6 weeks. A DNA PCR for HIV-1 should be done after delivery. In the newborns of HIV positive mothers, the infant's follow-up should be with a pediatric specialist in HIV care. Careful physical evaluation and HIV laboratory assessments are minimally performed at 6 weeks and 4 months.

If a woman has not had an HIV test done prior to delivery and falls into a high-risk category, the infant should be treated as if exposed to HIV. Start AZT prophylaxis and continue until HIV DNA PCR testing is done on the mother. If the mother still refuses HIV testing, then social work and perhaps a child's legal advocate should be consulted. If the child's mother is in the high-risk category and maternal HIV testing cannot be obtained, the full 6-week course should be given. If the mother wishes to ignore medical advice, the child welfare authorities should be consulted.

In the United States, mothers who are HIV positive should not breast-feed. In breast-feeding, the HIV-positive mother has a small, but not negligible, chance of giving HIV virus to the baby. In countries where safe formula and water are not available or where economics prevent formula-fed babies from receiving good nutrition, the ban on HIV-positive mothers breast-feeding is questionable. To save a child from HIV and then malnourish it, or have it die of severe gastroenteritis, is unconscionable.

HIV has become a major pandemic throughout the world, with every country reporting cases. The bulk of newly infected people reside in the Third World, particularly in Africa, Southeast Asia, India, and Latin America. In contrast, in the United States, the number of HIV-infected children younger than 13 years of age have accounted for only about 1% of HIV cases. With the medical regime described previously, over

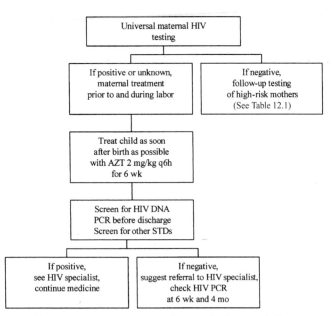

Figure 12.1   HIV—Preventing vertical transmission.

90% of these probable cases are currently being prevented in the United States. More than 8,500 cases of AIDS in children younger than 13 years of age have been reported to the CDC, and nearly half have already died of their disease. Minority groups, particularly African Americans and Hispanics, comprise the majority of children in the United States with HIV. Most of these children have acquired the disease by vertical transmission (mother to child), because the acquisition through blood and blood products has markedly decreased since the advent of scrupulous testing of the blood supply. In addition, the AIDS Clinical Trials Group protocol no. 076, which used Zidovudine (AZT) during pregnancy,

Table 12.1   High-risk mothers

- IV drug user
- Partner of IV drug user
- Sex worker
- Multiple sex partners
- Poor prenatal care
- Immigrant from endemic areas (e.g., Africa, SE Asia)

during labor, and for 6 weeks prophylaxis for the infant, originally resulted in a 67% reduction in perinatal transmission, and currently the numbers are even better. In those infants who have had proper maternal prophylaxis and 6 weeks of oral AZT following delivery, the likelihood of developing HIV disease after three negative PCRs is effectively zero. Congenital HIV has never been reported developing after a negative HIV test at 18 months of age.

The means to prevent HIV transmission from the mother to the infant is early recognition and prophylaxis. The American College of Obstetrics and Gynecology (ACOG) currently recommends that HIV testing be offered to all pregnant women. It appears that low maternal HIV loads and high CD4 cell counts decrease the risk of transmission to the infant. If proper control of the HIV virus is obtained during pregnancy, the prophylaxis for the infant during labor and postdelivery has been successful at preventing transmission in the vast majority of cases in the developed world.

At the time of birth, few if any infants have signs of HIV disease. They are, however, at risk for other sexually transmitted diseases (STDs) based on maternal risks. The diagnosis of HIV in the infant cannot rely on testing for HIV antibodies because of passive transmission of maternal HIV antibodies. The currently used test for the diagnosis of HIV infection in infants less than 6 months of age is a DNA PCR for HIV-1 or HIV culture. The PCR assay should not be performed on cord blood, because there is a possibility of maternal blood contamination of the sample. It is recommended that the infant undergo testing during the first few days of life, with a repeat HIV PCR at approximately 6 weeks of age and again at 4 months of age.

The standard prophylaxis for HIV is 2 mg per kg per dose q6h of AZT administered orally to the exposed infant as soon as possible after delivery (the IV route may be used if the oral route is not possible). The infant will continue this prophylaxis for 6 weeks until the second PCR is performed. At that visit, the infant will have a thorough physical examination performed, plotting height, weight, head circumference, developmental testing, complete blood cell count and chemistries, immunoglobulin, lymphocyte subsets, and the aforementioned PCR for HIV. The child will be placed on Bactrim for *Pneumocystitis carinii* prophylaxis, which will continue until the third HIV specialist visit at 4 months of age. During this third visit, all the labs done at the second visit are repeated, including PCR for HIV. If all the criteria for maternal and infant prophylaxis have been met and if all three HIV-1 RNA PCRs are negative, the child is discharged from further follow-up. Some centers are still continuing the practice of HIV enzyme-linked immunosorbent assay (ELISA) testing of the infant until the establishment of seronegativity. This is best accomplished at 3 to 4 month intervals beginning at approximately 9 months of age, and can coincide with well child visits. Approximately 50% of all infants who were originally HIV-1 ELISA seropositive are negative by 12 months of age. Almost all the rest of the infants become seronegative by 15 months of age.

Children do not manifest maternally derived HIV ELISA antibodies by 18 months of age.

In the developed world, AZT prophylaxis for mother and infant pairs has dramatically reduced the vertical transmission of HIV disease. Unfortunately, women even in the developed world still decline HIV testing during pregnancy or are not offered any. This leaves their children vulnerable to HIV transmission. Only further education and the development of a useful HIV vaccine, in addition to a potential cure for the disease, will make any impact on the staggering number of HIV-infected individuals in the world.

SUGGESTED READING

Mueller BU, Pizzo PA. Acquired immunodeficiency syndrome in the infant. In: Remington JA, Klein J, eds. *Infection of the fetus and newborn*. Philadelphia: WB Saunders, 2001:447–476.

Pickering LK, ed. *The red book,* 26th ed. Chicago: American Academy of Pediatrics, 2003.

CHAPTER 13

Hepatitis and Other Liver Inflammations

Gary A. Emmett and Sue Jue

Almost all diseases cause some liver dysfunction in the newborn, but this chapter concerns primary liver diseases and diseases whose presenting signs or symptoms are liver inflammation.

The following two diseases of the liver result in unconjugated hyperbilirubinimia. *Crigler-Najjar syndrome,* a defect of one of the microsomal enzymes that conjugate bilirubin (bilirubin uridine diphosphate glucuronosyltransferase, UGT, to be specific) is extremely rare but, in its type I phenotype, it can cause serum indirect bilirubins of greater than 20 mg/dL very quickly. It often results in kernicterus. Diagnosis is by lack of bilirubin diglucuronide in the bile.

The *Gilbert syndrome* is usually quite benign and is rarely expressed until puberty when mild unconjugated hyperbilirubinemia occurs in times of fasting or stress. It is a defect in the expression of the UGT enzyme involving one or two extra TAs (thyrosine-adenosine) in the TATA box of the DNA of that enzyme. Up to 10% of humans have this altered gene expression. The importance of the Gilbert syndrome is that in newborns with high bilirubins, it can make the problem much worse. A positive family history will make the practitioner more wary.

Most liver inflammations result in conjugated hyperbilirubinemia. The most common causes in the well nursery are listed in Table 13.1. Infection by bacterial sepsis (Chapter 9) and in the TORCH syndromes (Chapter 11) are covered in their own chapters, but hepatitis B and C are covered in the paragraphs that follow.

Hepatitis B prevention is one of the primary goals of the well nursery. Hepatitis B is endemic in East Asia, and before vaccination in the nursery was started, over 16,000 babies in the United States developed perinatal hepatitis B each year. Perinatal disease is rarely acquired prenatally (less than 2% of the cases), but both delivery and the months immediately after birth have high rates of transmission (up to 90% in mothers with both HbsAg and HbeAg positive). One of the confusing questions is: "What do all the antigens and antibodies mean in terms of the disease's infectivity?" Table 13.2 tries to explicate this dilemma.

In most cases, there are no acute symptoms in perinatal hepatitis B. The only safe way to protect against hepatitis B is to give the vaccine while the child is in the hospital. If not immunized, up to 90% of children exposed to hepatitis B–positive mothers will become carriers.

Table 13.1   Causes of conjugated hyperbilirubin in the newborn

Infections
    TORCH infections
    Bacterial sepsis
    Hepatitis B
    Hepatitis C
Genetic disorders
    Alpha$_1$ Antitrypsin deficiency (also called Alpha$_1$ Antiproteinase deficiency)
    Cystic fibrosis
    Galactosemia (the most common genetic disorder in the first week of life)
    Hypothyroidism
Obstructions of the bile system and the gastrointestinal tract
    Biliary atresia
    Choledochal cysts
    Small bowel obstructions and/or duplications

Later, 25% of the exposed untreated children will develop liver cancer as adults.

Figure 13.1 is a visual representation of the pathway described here for treating babies born to HbsAg-positive, negative, and unknown mothers. If the mother is *hepatitis B–positive,* the only method that achieves the full measure of protection for the child is the following:

- Hepatitis B vaccine within 12 hours of birth (preferably immediately after birth), with a repeat in at least 28 days and no more than 35 days

- *And* hepatitis B–specific immunoglobulin (both 0.5 cc IM) within 7 days.

In mothers with unknown hepatitis B status, do not hesitate to give the vaccine immediately, but wait for the costly and rare immunoglobulin until the mother's hepatitis B is available, as long as the wait is under 7 days. See Table 13.3.

Black Box Warning!

In many practices, the second hepatitis B is incorporated into the combined DaPT/IPV/Hep B immunization and given at 2 months of age. This is not safe for babies who have hepatitis B–positive mothers. The first booster must be given in 28 to 35 days. There is no need to change any other routine. Extra hepatitis B shots do not cause harm.

Table 13.2   Differentiation of hepatitis B blood tests

Presence of HBeAg implies infectivity
Presence of Anti-HBeAg does not eliminate infectivity

Disease State ▶ Blood Markers ▲	HBsAg	Anti-HBs	HBeAg	Anti-HBe	Anti-HBc	IgM Anti-HBc
Vaccinated	+	+	–	–	–	–
New disease	+	–	–/+	+	+	+
Chronic Carrier	+	–/+	+	+	+	–
Inactive old disease	+	+	–	–	+	–

HBsAg	Hepatitis B surface antigen
Anti-HBs	Antibody to hepatitis surface antigen
HBeAg	Hepatitis B E antigen
Anti-HBe	Antibody to hepatitis B E antigen
Anti-HBc	Antibody to hepatitis B core antigen (the IgG antibody)
IgM Anti-HBc	IgM Antibody to hepatitis B core antigen

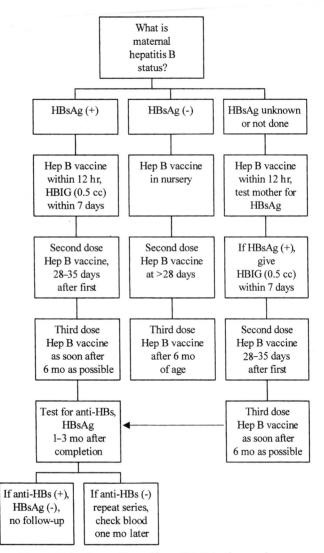

Figure 13.1   Prevention of hepatitis B in the newborn.

Table 13.3   Prevention of hepatitis B in the newborn

Both hepatitis B vaccine and hepatitis B immunoglobulin are 0.5-cc IM injections

If mother is hepatitis B (−)	• Vaccine after birth	F/U booster after 28 days
If mother is hepatitis B (+)	• Vaccine within 12 hr • Hepatitis B immunoglobulin within 1 wk	F/U booster 28–35 days old
If mother is hepatitis B unknown	• Vaccine within 12 hr • Determine mother's hepatitis B status • Hepatitis B immunoglobulin within 1 wk if needed	F/U booster according to mother's hepatitis B status

Breast-feeding in hepatitis B–positive mothers does not increase the child's risk of acquiring disease from the mother.

Hepatitis C–positive mothers constitute about 1 to 2% of all pregnancies. This is the same percentage as in the general population. About 5% of their babies will acquire antibodies to hepatitis C. Symptoms are rare, and less than 20% of the children will be jaundiced. There is no prophylaxis that is currently known to be effective. Breast-feeding is acceptable as long as the breasts are not cracked and bleeding.

Alpha₁-antitrypsin deficiency is a recessive disorder that is found primarily in Americans of northern European descent. Many variant genes have been found in the genotype of this protease inhibitor, but the ZZ genotype is the variant that causes severe liver disease in the child and fatal emphysema in the adult (especially in smokers). About one in six people with the ZZ genotype will develop a direct hyperbilirubinemia in the first few weeks of life. If left unchecked, children would die of progressive cirrhosis. Gene replacement may be in the future, and protein replacement will help the lung disease, but not the liver disease. In severe cases, the only solution presently is liver transplantation.

Cystic fibrosis is a recessive disorder with a defect in the cystic fibrosis transmembrane regulator (CFTR). CFTR allows the body to secrete chloride and water at the same time, so that secretions stay moist and do not cause clogging of passageways. Over a thousand variant genes have been found in this disorder, which subsequently has a wide range of expression. In the newborn, direct hyperbilirubinemia, meconium plug with delayed stooling, and persistent dark nasal discharge are the most common expressions.

61

Table 13.4   The signs and symptoms of galactosemia

- Lethargy
- GI disturbance (especially vomiting)
- Failure to thrive (usually lose weight)
- Kidney dysfunction
- Dehydration
- Direct hyperbilirubinemia with liver dysfunction and clotting defects
- Bacterial sepsis 7–21 days after birth with gram-negative organisms

Galactosemia is the general term for defects in three different enzymes in the metabolic pathway that converts galactose to glucose-1-phosphate. Galactose is a breakdown product of lactose (milk sugar) that is found in almost all mammalian milk. Therefore, if a child is on formula derived from either mother's milk or cow's milk after birth, the child will get progressively ill over time. In the case of classic galactosemia, the defect is in galactose 1-phosphate uridyltransferase. The multiple problems that result from the accumulation of galactose 1-phosphate in the tissue are listed in Table 13.4. Table 13.5 lists the results of absent or inadequate treatment.

In short, if a newborn is irritable, lethargic, intolerant of feeding (usually with vomiting), and/or not gaining weight, check the urine for glucose and other reducing substances. If the glucose is negative (Clinistix) and the other reducing substance is positive (Clinitest), then galactosemia is likely. Using a nonlactose formula resolves all acute problems, but the lack of UDP-galactose in the tissues may cause subtle long-term problems such as learning disabilities.

Congenial _hypothryroidism_ may result from absence or dysgenesis of the thyroid, from an enzyme defect in the hormonal cascade, or from environmental disturbance (high-dose iodine perinatally, transplacental absorption of antithyroid drugs, and maternal antithyroid antibodies). Its occurrence is 1 in 3,000 to 4,000 births, which makes it the most likely serious condition found with the newborn screening program. If untreated, it will result in poor growth and severe developmental delay in both mind and body.

Table 13.5   The systemic results of untreated or inadequately treated galactosemia

- Sepsis
- Cataracts
- Mental retardation
- Cirrhosis
- Myopathy
- Death

Table 13.6   Symptoms of congenital hypothyroidism

- Prolonged direct hyperbilirubinemia
- Poor temperature maintenance
- Poor feeding
- Poor growth
- Constipation
- Hoarseness
- Umbilical hernia
- Poor interaction with others

If hypothyroidism is suspected (see Table 13.6), then the newborn screen should be checked with a low serum total T_4 (8–14 mcg/dL first week in a full-term infant) and a very high thyroid-stimulating hormone (TSH, thyrotropin; >13 mlU/mL in the first week of life). Therapy is L-thyroxine (having a consistent brand is important, because bioavailability varies with the product) at 10 to 15 micrograms per kilogram once daily. Hypothyroidism is a difficult disease both to diagnose and to treat, and an expert in pediatric endocrinology should be consulted after abnormal tests are found.

Biliary atresia usually presents as a progressive prolonged direct hyperbilirubinemia sometime in the first month of life. This progressive obliteration of the lumens of biliary ducts is probably postintrauterine viral infection. Autoimmune and insufficient vascularization have also been suggested as causes, but none have been proven. The occurrence is about one in 10,000 births. Acholic stools are common, and the liver can be enlarged. A liver biopsy and/or an operative cholangiogram are needed for definitive diagnosis. If diagnosed early, a Kasai procedure (a hepatoportoenterostomy) may be life saving. Unfortunately, in up to 90% of children with biliary atresia, a liver transplant is needed.

To diagnose and treat the multiple rare causes of distal bile blockage such as duplicate small bowel or a pseudocyst of the pancreas, ultrasound and MRI imaging are indicated. Once the cause is established, then a qualified surgeon can treat many of these lesions.

SUGGESTED READING

Schwartz MW, ed. *The 5-minute pediatric consult,* 2nd ed. Philadelphia: Lippincott, 2000. On page 180 under Laboratory Aids, there is an excellent list of all the procedures one may need to definitively diagnose direct hyperbilirubinemia.

Pickering LK, ed. *The red book,* 26th ed. Chicago: American Academy of Pediatrics, 2003.

CHAPTER 14
Varicella (Chicken Pox)

Gary A. Emmett

Exposure to varicella during pregnancy may be fatal to both mother and child and should never be taken lightly.

Varicella (chicken pox) in the first few days of life may be fatal to a newborn. Any maternal exposure to varicella, especially late in the pregnancy, requires aggressive medical intervention. Varicella is caused by the herpes-zoster virus and has a primary presentation of fever and a papulovesicular rash. The classic rash of chicken pox consists of clear vesicles on an irregular red base, which is familiarly known as "a dew drop on a rose petal." In the past, most cases of varicella in the United States occurred in children less than 10 years old, but with the rapid expansion of the vaccine program, the number of children with chicken pox has fallen greatly, although adult cases have fallen to a lesser degree. Some adults, including pregnant women, did not acquire immunity from childhood disease and remain susceptible.

During the primary infection, the varicella-zoster virus (VZV) establishes itself in dorsal root ganglia, and can later manifest itself as herpes zoster (shingles). Herpes zoster is characterized by a painful papulovesicular rash usually localized in one or, at most, two dermatones. Both active varicella and shingles cases may transmit VZV to other human beings. Humans are infected when the virus comes in contact with the mucosa of the upper respiratory tract or the conjunctivae. Varicella has a high index of infectivity and, though contact person-to-person spread is by far the most common mode of infection, it can occasionally spread by airborne particles. Unfortunately, in utero infection can also occur by transplancental passage of virus during active maternal varicella and, rarely, with maternal shingles. The incubation period for mother-to-fetus infection is 10 to 21 days. Spread of infection can occur from one to two days before the onset of rash until all lesions are crusted over.

Although generally considered to be a benign childhood illness in the United States, severe complications can occur even in immuno-competent patients. Bacterial superinfection of skin lesions (primarily through group A beta-hemolytic streptococcus), pneumonia, arthritis, hepatitis, cerebellar ataxia, encephalitis, or glomerulonephritis may occur in normal children. Complications occur more often and are more serious in immunocompromised patients, and are also worse if the patient is past puberty. Fetal infection after maternal varicella during the first or early second trimester of pregnancy can occasionally result in the congenital varicella syndrome, which is characterized by limb atrophy, scarring of the skin on the extremities, central nervous system

Part III
The Well Nursery

Hyperbilirubinemia in the Well Nursery

Gary A. Emmett

The only purpose for following and treating jaundice in the newborn is preventing bilirubin encephalopathy. All effects of jaundice appear to be completely reversible if cell death does not occur.

Kernicterus (bilirubin encephalopathy) is not a disease of the past. Bilirubin encepahalopathy still occurs, though much more rarely than in the past. This chapter gives parameters for the treatment of neonatal jaundice, explains the pattern of both nonpathologic and pathologic jaundice in the well newborn, and describes bilirubin's pathologic consequences. Included in this chapter are the differential diagnosis of unconjugated hyperbilirubinemia and a pathway to prevent harm to the babies born in your nursery. The pathway is shown in Fig. 15.1.

Bilirubin is an end product of red cell destruction. It serves as an antioxidant that prevents RNA mutation. Eventually, the body must eliminate the excess bilirubin. The bilirubin traverses the bloodstream in a one-to-one relationship with albumin, is absorbed into the hepatocyte via the X and Y proteins, is conjugated by the microsomal enzymes, and is expelled as direct bilirubin via the biliary tract and eventually the gut. Table 15.1 presents bilirubin definitions.

Normally, 90% or more of bilirubin is excreted via stool, but visible light at 440 Angstrom units (blue) will cause bilirubin in blood vessels near the skin to undergo a steric change and become the relatively water-soluble *photobilirubin*, which can be excreted through the urine.

In a normal newborn, there is a biphasic bilirubin curve with a low peak at about 5 to 6 hours of age and another peak 2 to 4 days later. The curves are different for bottle- and breast-fed babies, with the maximum for bottle-fed babies occurring at 48 to 60 hours, whereas in breast-fed babies, the maximum is between 100 and 120 hours (see Fig. 15.2). It has been shown that predicting maximum bilirubin depends primarily on the age of the child at the time of the measurement and the level of bilirubin in the bloodstream at that time.

From the early 1950s studies of hyperbilirubinemia in Rh disease, we know that bilirubin encephalopathy is exceedingly rare in healthy full-term newborns with unconjugated bilirubins of less than 25 mg/dL, but not all babies in the well baby nursery are full term. In the

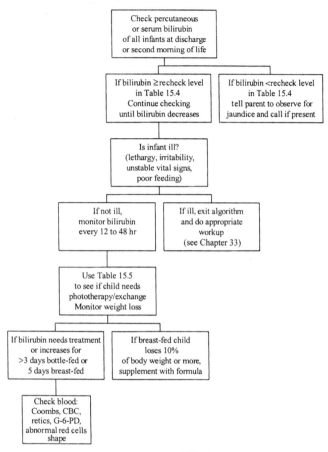

Figure 15.1   Hyperbilirubinemia.

United States in 1999, the rate of babies born at 36 weeks of gestation or less was up to 11% of all births; many of the 34- to 37-week newborns without obvious problems may go to the well baby nursery and not to an intensive care unit. It is the "well" borderline premature infants who are most likely to get brain damage from bilirubin encephalopathy, because their average bilirubin concentrations are higher and occur at later times than the 40-week-gestation baby. Borderline premature gestation is one of the more important factors in bilirubin encephalopathy, as can be seen from Table 15.2.

The exact pathophysiology of bilirubin encephalopathy is not known, but in children with permanent damage, there is deep yellow staining of

Table 15.1   Definitions

Bilirubin is assumed to be *unconjugated bilirubin* (also called indirect bilirubin) unless stated otherwise. Unconjugated bilirubin is not water soluble and is toxic to brain tissue in high concentration.

Conjugated bilirubin (also called direct bilirubin and bilirubin glucuronide or diglucuronide) is water soluble and is benign. Unfortunately, if the conjugated bilirubin spends too much time in the gut, the enterohepatic circulation will reabsorb and deconjugate the bilirubin, which will reenter the blood stream and reattach to albumin if available.

Photobilirubin is a steric isomer of bilirubin that is relatively water soluble, but it is in an unstable energy state and will revert to bilirubin within an hour or so if not excreted.

the basal ganglia and various brainstem nuclei. This damage is apparent on a magnetic resonance imaging (MRI) scan.

A child with bilirubin encephalopathy starts with sepsislike symptoms of lethargy, poor feeding, and loss of the Moro reflex as the excess unconjugated bilirubin attaches to the nerve terminals. The second phase begins with the bilirubin infiltrating the cell and attaching to the microsomes, after which the child becomes "septic" with poor reflexes, high-pitched and weak cry, and even respiratory distress because of poor respiratory effort. As the bilirubin seeps through the entire neuron, clinically a shrill cry and even retrocollis (backward arching of neck) and opisthotonus (backward arching of trunk) may result. During this third phase, the process becomes irreversible. Finally, there is neuronal destruction with pyknosis, and over the next 3 years, there is a constantly changing set of neurological signs with both hypotonia and hypertonia, mild to severe developmental delay, and seizures ending in

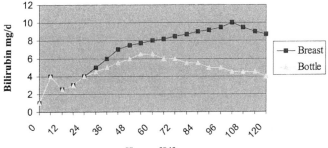

Figure 15.2   **Physiologic jaundice in full-term newborns.**

Table 15.2   Risk factors for bilirubin encephalopathy in the well baby nursery

---

- Jaundice in the first 24 hr of life
- Visible jaundice before discharge
- Previous sibling with jaundice
- Gestation 38 wk or less
- Exclusively breast-feeding
- Dark skin color, especially East Asian race
- Bruising including cephalohematoma
- Maternal age >than 25 yr
- Male sex

---

choreoathetosis, seizures, stiffness, poor speech, high-frequency hearing loss, and inability to raise the eyes upward. Auditory evoked response (AER) is an excellent measure for following bilirubin encephalopathy, being both sensitive and specific to this toxin.

A newborn may become jaundiced through one or more of the following three processes: Red cells are too rapidly destroyed, the body cannot properly conjugate bilirubin, or the gut cannot eliminate conjugated bilirubin quickly enough to prevent reabsorption via the enterohepatic circulation. The conjugated bilirubin becomes reabsorbed through the enterohepatic circulation. During enterohepatic reabsorption, the bilirubin is unconjugated again. In general, erythrocyte destruction results in unconjugated hyperbilirubinemia (more than 90% of bilirubin is unconjugated), and processing and elimination problems result in conjugated hyperbilirubinemia. The differential diagnosis of unconjugated hyperbilirubinemia is found in Figure 15.3. The differential diagnosis of conjugated bilirubinemia is found in Chapter 13.

The most common causes for increased production of bilirubin are listed in Table 15.3. Many authors differentiate breast-milk jaundice from breast-feeding jaundice, because breast-milk jaundice is caused primarily by the direct effect of the breast milk on liver uptake of the bilirubin, whereas breast-feeding jaundice is caused by an inadequate milk supply in the mother, producing dehydration and reduced stooling. Trauma is often ignored, but is a major source of the hemolysis that produces an excess amount of bilirubin. Isoimmunization of the red cells occurs when the mother has the null state at her red cell antigenic site while the baby does not. Because ABO isoimmunization is relatively mild and Rh disease is largely prevented with the use of RhoGAM, four of the minor red cell antigens, Kell, Duffy, Lewis, and MNO, are now the most common cause of erythroblastosis fetalis. G-6-PD deficiency is most frequently found in the United States in African American males. Many believe it often leads to kernicterus.

Traditionally, the night nurse uses visual diagnosis to choose which newborns receive early morning bilirubins. The practitioners use visual

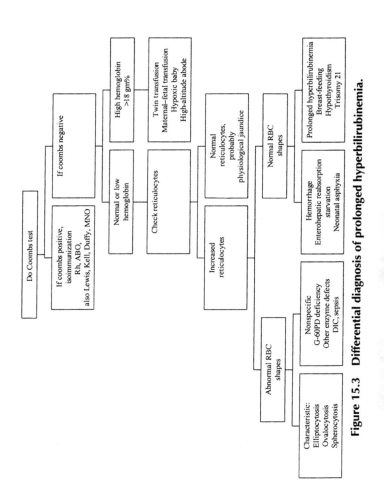

Figure 15.3   Differential diagnosis of prolonged hyperbilirubinemia.

Table 15.3   Causes of hyperbilirubinemia in the neonate

1. Normal physiologic jaundice
2. Breast-feeding jaundice/breast-milk jaundice
3. Trauma: bruising, cephalohematomas, facial suffusion, intracranial bleeding
4. Isoimmmunization of the red cell, primarily caused by ABO, Rh, Kell, Duffy, Lewis, and MNO
5. G-6-PD deficiency
6. Congenital erythrocyte wall defects (ovalocytosis, spherocytosis, elliptocytosis)
7. Sepsis

diagnosis to add more on their rounds in the morning. This process is problematic for two reasons:

- It misses some icteric babies who are not noticeably jaundiced.

- It delays the discharge of the babies chosen to receive bilirubins in the morning.

Interference with visual diagnosis of jaundice may be caused by poor lighting, hospital color schemes, and babies of color. To avoid missing any babies with jaundice, some institutions simply check the serum bilirubin on all 2-day-old infants (or any discharges less than 2 days). This option is very safe, but it may be expensive. A third alternative that has recently become available is to use a percutaneous bilirubinometer on every 2-day-old infant (and any discharges before 2 days). By matching the age of the baby to the age range in Table 15.4, the practitioner can choose those who need follow-up bilirubins.

This pathway may become standard when the per capita cost of the percutaneous readings decreases to significantly below the cost of

Table 15.4   Bilirubin follow-up decisions

Age (hr)	Discharge if bilirubin is	Follow-up bilirubin within 48 hr
<24	<8	All babies
24–36	<11	>7
37–48	<13	>8
49–60	<14	>9
61–72	<15	>10
>72	<16	>12 and still rising

a serum bilirubin level, especially if the bilirubinometers become so accurate on all skin colors that no serum bilirubins are necessary. A wise discharge strategy is to tell each new mother to check the color of the baby in the sunlight every day for the first week and call the baby's primary care practitioner if the child appears to have gotten markedly more yellow.

Actual treatment of hyperbilirubinemia starts with simply increasing the oral intake of the child and placing the child in the sunlight. The two forms of medical intervention were both introduced in the 1950s: exchange transfusion and phototherapy. Exchange transfusion was extremely common in earlier decades when Rh disease was still extant, but now is restricted to the realm of neonatologists and should not be done in the well baby nursery under any circumstances. Phototherapy can be delivered to the baby with many different instruments, but they are all concentrated on the same physical constants: delivering the largest possible flux of 440-Angstrom light to the largest possible skin area of the infant. The bilirubin blanket of dim blue lights at the actual skin level has made doing phototherapy at home practical, but is safe and useful only in the mildest cases. In general, the more lights there are and the closer those lights are to the infant, the more effective is the phototherapy. Also, new lamps are almost always better than older lamps, and the flux of the lamps should be tested regularly. Safety measures include covering the infant's eyes and preventing overheating of the infant. Babies under phototherapy act as if they were spending too much time on the beach: They are mildly cranky, sleepy, and have loose stools.

The approach to the parents in discussing hyperbilirubinemia is crucial in preventing physiologic and psychologic damage to the child, caused by the treatment of this physiologic process. The practitioner in the newborn nursery must be firm but warm in discussing the problem of hyperbilirubinemia. Many mothers become guilt wracked when told that their antibodies are harming their child because of isoimmunization problems. Even more mothers are dissuaded from breast-feeding because of the child losing too much weight or having a high bilirubin. The practitioner must be supportive and convince the mother that breast-feeding is not harming her child. Invoking guilt is counterproductive and must be avoided. At the same time, supplementing with formula to avoid dehydration is not evil and should be encouraged if it allows the child to avoid medical intervention.

Table 15.5, indications for hyperbilirubin intervention, is a simplified guide to starting phototherapy. These are suggestions for the full-term well infant, but many practitioners start therapy at lower levels, depending on other sociologic and physiologic problems. If phototherapy is indicated, it should be used immediately and with a maximum flux of 440-Angstrom light so that an exchange transfusion may be avoided.

C H A P T E R   16
Physical Examination
J. Lindsey Lane

The physical examination is the basis of all primary care. It is often relegated to a minor role in this age of MRIs and PET scans, but more knowledge can be gained in less time from a simple physical examination than almost any other means of diagnosing the child.

INTERPRETING THE VITAL SIGNS

Table 16.1 lists vital signs for the newborn. These values must be measured and recorded on a chart.

Temperature is often misunderstood. A reading of 98.6°F is not normal temperature, it is the average temperature of an adult, also expressed as an even number in Celsius (37°C). In the well nursery, babies should be above 97° within an hour or two of birth, and should not have temperatures measured from the skin or axilla of 100°F or more.

The average *heart rate* of a newborn infant is 120 beats per minute (bpm), but this may range from 80 to 160 bpm depending on whether the baby is in deep sleep or very active. Brief depression of the heart rate to 70 and elevation to 200 or slightly above may be seen in some normal newborns.

Very large (greater than 4.5 kg) or postdate (more than 41 weeks of gestation) infants often have periodic *bradycardia* (less than 90 beats per minute) during sleep, but the heart rate returns to normal on stimulation. Newborns who are persistently bradycardic need evaluation by a physician. Accurate identification of the cause will guide therapy; many times a consultation with a pediatric cardiologist is appropriate. Some of the common causes of isolated bradycardia and appropriate interventions are listed in Table 16.2.

Tachycardia (more than 160 beats per minute) may be caused by hyperthermia. Infants delivered by a mother who is febrile will initially also be febrile, as will infants who have been overheated in an isolette or on a radiant warmer. The tachycardia should resolve when the body temperature of the infant returns to normal. Sepsis, hypovolemia, and heart failure must be considered if the tachycardia persists. More rarely, tachycardia may be caused by congenital hyperthyroidism or by the action of maternally ingested thyroid hormone. Maternal drugs even as

Table 16.1   Vital signs must be measured and recorded on chart

Temperature	98°F–99.5°F (36.8°C–37.5°C) rectal
Heart rate	80–160 per min (brief periods down to 70 and up to 200 acceptable)
Respiratory rate	30–80 per min first day without distress, 30–60 thereafter
Blood pressure	Systolic/diastolic—5th to 95th percentiles for 40 wk gestation
	Day 1 45–65/25–40
	Day 3 50–70/30–45
	Day 5 55–75/33–48
Length, weight	See Figs. 17.1 and 17.3
Head circumference	See Figs. 17.2 and 17.4
Gestational age	See Fig. 17.5

Table 16.2   Causes of bradycardia in newborns

Cause	Evaluation/Management
Hypothermia	Warm infant, consider sepsis (if cannot warm)
Maternal medications:	
Magnesium (most common)	Mg^{++} level, supportive care
Digoxin	Digoxin level, Fab fragments
Calcium channel blockers	Calcium chloride
Beta blockers	Isoproterenol
Increasing intracranial pressure	Head ultrasound
Acute (e.g., intracranial bleeding)	CT scan
	May need mechanical ventilation
Subacute (e.g., hydrocephalus)	May need surgery
Hypothyroidism in mother or infant	T4, thyrotropin thyroid hormone replacement
Complete (3rd degree) atrioventricular (AV) block associated with congenital heart disease	Cardiology consult
	Ventricular pacing
	Also associated with maternal lupus or other CT disease
Postdates, large for gestational age (LGA)	Stimulate to resolve
Neonatal asphyxia	Supportive care

Table 16.3   Causes of tachycardia in the well nursery

Cause	Evaluation/Management
Hyperthermia	Cool infant
	Consider sepsis (if fever persists)
Hypovolemia	Fluid resuscitation
Maternal medications or drugs (caffeine, nicotine, herbs such as lobeline)	Await resolution
Hyperthyroidism in mother or infant	T4, thyrotropin
Conduction abnormalities	ECG, cardiology consult
Supraventricular tachypnea (SVT)	Adenosine (acutely)
	Digitalization
Premature ventricular contractions (PVCs; multiform or runs)	Lidocaine, echocardiogram
Ventricular tachycardia	Direct current cardioversion
	Long-term beta blockers
Heart failure/congenital heart disease (CHD)	Digoxin
	Lasix
Persistent patent ductus arteriosis (PDA)	Prostaglandin E1
	Surgery

common as nicotine, herbs, over-the-counter (OTC) cold preparations, and caffeine have been known to cause tachycardia in the breast-fed infant. See Table 16.3 for causes of tachycardia in the well nursery.

Many *arrhythmias* can occur in the newborn nursery. Premature atrial contractions (PAC) occur in up to one third of normal infants. Nonsinus rhythm is also seen in up to one third of infants; the most common causes are junctional or nodal rhythm, followed by premature ventricular contractions (PVC) in up to 13% normal infants and supraventricular tachycardia (SVT) in up to 4% of normal infants.

A junctional (nodal) rhythm may be idiopathic or associated with congenital heart defect (CHD), increased vagal tone, or digitalis toxicity. If the infant with a junctional rhythm is asymptomatic, no treatment is necessary; however, if the infant has symptoms from the bradycardia, atropine or electrical pacing may be needed. Nodal premature beats and nodal escape beats are benign, but may be associated with digitalis toxicity. It is important to remember that pharyngeal and nasal suctioning will often cause increases in vagal tone and secondary bradycardia.

PVCs are usually benign, but they can be associated with CHD, myocarditis, cardiomyopathy, cardiac tumors, hyperkalemia, asphyxia, stimulant drugs, and long QT syndrome. Multiform PVCs and runs of PVCs are more likely to have a pathological cause and to need intervention.

SVT may be caused by abnormal intrinsic cardiac conduction pathways and more rarely by myocarditis, thyrotoxicosis, and structural heart defects.

The various cardiac rhythms and conduction disturbances must be differentiated from each other on electrocardiogram (ECG). An echocardiogram often aids in revealing structural defects. Evaluation and management should be done in consultation with a pediatric cardiologist.

The newborn *respiratory rate* is usually in the 40s or 50s. A rate greater than 60 requires evaluation by the attending, as it may indicate sepsis or pulmonary pathology. A transcutaneous pulse oximetry determination is a helpful addition to the vital signs. If the infant has good oxygenation and otherwise looks well, the tachypnea is most likely due to a difficult transition, so-called transient tachypnea of the newborn (TTN), which should resolve in under 6 hours with no intervention. Hypothermia and hyperthermia may also cause tachypnea that will resolve over an hour or two as the infant is warmed or cooled. If the newborn has risk factors for sepsis or has other abnormal findings such as a low glucose and/or appears sick, a chest radiograph should be done together with other laboratory investigation, and appropriate treatment should be instituted. (See Chapter 32.)

Blood pressure (BP) is measured using the Dinamapp and an appropriately sized disposable plastic cuff. Many nurseries take blood pressures in all four extremities. If there is a markedly lower BP in the lower extremities than the upper, it may indicate an aortic coarctation. If the coarctation is preductal, the infant may go into heart failure as soon as the ductus arteriosus fully closes, and timely intervention with administration of prostaglandin E1 will be helpful.

Accurate measurements of the *weight, length,* and *head circumference* are central to the care of the newborn. Remember that newborns do not always cooperate while being measured, and mistakes are made. If the height (especially), weight, or head circumference seems wrong, remeasure. Assessment of the gestational age of the baby (see Chapter 17) is needed to correlate the height, weight, and head size with other clinical observations. Because the expected date of confinement (EDC) may not be accurate, use the Ballard scale (see Tables 17.1 and 17.2) to assess the baby's gestational age in weeks. The practitioner can then see if the infant's weight is small, appropriate, or large for gestational age (SGA, AGA, LGA), and using the head circumference, can classify the infant as microcephalic, normocephalic, or macrocephalic.

Any infant with abnormal growth parameters causes the practitioner to delve into the history and review other parts of the physical examination to discover the cause. Remember that abnormal means more than two standard deviations from the mean, and abnormal is not necessarily pathologic.

THE NEWBORN PHYSICAL EXAMINATION

After examination of the vital signs, the practitioner makes an overall observation of the infant. Looking at the infant as a single impression is called a *gestalt*. The human eye and brain are remarkable in their ability to identify patterns of normality and alert us when the *gestalt* is "different." If we look at a newborn and get an impression of "pathologic," we can then proceed to identify the specific features that gave us that impression. This is how we identify infants with trisomy 21 (Down syndrome) or Rubinstein-Taybi syndrome, for example. After the overall observation has given us an impression of normal or abnormal, we can move on to touch the baby and examine the specific organ systems.

Many examiners begin the newborn examination with the *cardiorespiratory systems*, because these systems can be difficult to examine if the infant is crying. Color changes in the newborn skin may be confused with cardiac problems. Many infants with facial suffusion (ecchymotic face secondary to a tight nuchal cord or a face presentation) may be thought initially to be cyanotic until completely examined. Sometimes, because of the vascular instability of newborns, you will see acrocyanosis (blue hands and/or feet), perioral duskiness, or a diffuse reticular (netlike) pink and red pattern of the skin. All of these are normal variants that require no intervention.

Murmurs are very common in the newborn. There are several types of innocent murmurs that may be heard in the newborn period. These include:

- ductal murmur, as the ductus arteriosus completes its closure;

- tricuspid insufficiency murmur, as insignificant amounts of blood leak through the tricuspid valve; and

- peripheral pulmonic stenosis murmur, where the blood creates audible turbulence as it flows through the pulmonic valve and the pulmonary vascular bed.

None of these murmurs is associated with any other findings (such as an abnormal splitting of the second heart sound), and they are all systolic and soft. If these murmurs persist, or if the infant seems ill in any way, a pediatric cardiology consultation is advised. The precordium should be palpated for thrills or heaves, and the presence and volume of the peripheral pulses should be assessed. Remember to check the inguinal pulses daily, because, until the ductus arteriosus closes, they may seem normal even in the presence of aortic coarctation.

The breath sounds can be evaluated next. It is unusual to hear an abnormality in the absence of an increased respiratory rate or other sign of respiratory distress. Some newborns have nasal congestion that causes transmitted upper airway noises to be heard with the stethoscope. If the nasal congestion is severe, the infant may be in respiratory distress,

81

as newborns are obligate nose breathers. Gently clearing the mucus with a bulb suction syringe is often all that is needed. The caregiver should be taught how to do this. It is important to make sure that unilateral choanal atresia is not the cause of the noisy breathing. Test for unilateral choanal atresia by passing a catheter through each nostril into the hypopharynx. Some newborns make a noise called "stridor." This is a characteristic inspiratory sound that is caused by a narrowing of the airway somewhere between the pharynx and the bifurcation of the trachea. There are several causes, some more common than others. Any infant with stridor needs immediate evaluation.

After examining the cardiorespiratory system, one starts at the top of the *head* and examines the baby down to the toes. By measuring and plotting the head circumference on the growth chart at the appropriate gestational age, the practitioner will have already decided whether the baby's head is normal in size. It is quite common for the head to show signs of trauma from the delivery and to be somewhat distorted in shape, what is called "molding," from having passed through the birth canal. The suture lines will be overriding, and the anterior and posterior (if present) fontanels will be distorted, compared to how they will appear 24 hours or so later. There may be soft tissue edema (caput) and some-times a subperiostial accumulation of blood, especially on the parietal bone (cephalohematoma). A caput generally resolves very quickly, but a cephalohematoma may take several weeks to resolve as the blood organizes and is eventually resorbed. It is important to distinguish these benign swellings from the more serious encephaloceles or meningoceles or soft tissue swellings that overlie a skull fracture. If a fracture is significantly depressed, then it will need to be surgically elevated. Scalp abrasions may be noted and are more likely if instrumentation such as a vacuum extraction or forceps has been used to deliver the head. If an internal lead was applied to monitor the fetal heart rate prior to delivery, a break in the integrity of the dermis will be apparent at the site of application of the lead. Any break in the skin should be serially followed for signs of infection, and it may be wise to apply topical antibiotic ointment prophylactically.

It is important to make sure that the *eyes* are not too far apart (hyper-telorism) or too close together (hypotelorism). The range for normal intercanthal distance is 1.5 to 2.6 cm. Also check that the eyelid(s) do not droop (ptosis) and that eye shape and palpebral fissure width are normal. The globes should be examined. It is quite common to see half-moon-shaped subconjunctival hemorrhages that occur secondary to the rapid change in pressure as the head is delivered. It is essential that the eyes are examined using an ophthalmoscope to make sure that the lens has no opacities (cataracts) and that the cornea is not cloudy (congenital glaucoma). To make sure that the rest of the visual axis as far as the retina is unobstructed, the red reflex should be elicited in both eyes. Remember that the red reflex is often orange and orange/gray.

The *ears* are examined to make sure that they are normal in shape, size, and position, and that the external auditory canal is patent.

Low-set ears are a common feature in many genetic syndromes. If less than 10% of the pinna is above a line drawn horizontally from the medial canthus of the eye to the occiput, then the ears are low set. A very common abnormality is to find small preauricular pits or tags. Very often another family member has the same finding. It is important to remember that occasionally these branchial cleft remnants are associated with deafness.

Some nasal congestion and mucus are common, and often babies sneeze reflexively as a means of clearing the *nose*. The nasal septum should be in midline. Rarely, there is choanal atresia where the nasal passage has not completely canalized. If atresia is bilateral, the infant will be in respiratory distress.

Two very important reflexes associated with the *mouth*, the sucking reflex and the rooting reflex, should be elicited. The hard and soft palates should be inspected and palpated for clefts and the gums examined for cysts and the rare finding of a natal tooth. Sometimes you may note a "tongue tie," where the lingual frenulum seems very short or tight. The tight frenulum is usually not associated with future speech problems, but some breast-feeding experts state that tongue tie can interfere with effective sucking in the breast-fed infant. The symmetry of the mouth when the baby is crying is important, especially if there has been a forceps delivery, as the facial nerve may have been damaged, as it passes through the parotid gland.

The range of motion of the *neck* should be tested to ensure that there is no torticollis. Most commonly, this condition is due to a unilaterally shortened sternocleidomastoid muscle. Sometimes a firm "tumor" of the muscle can be palpated. Usually, if the parents perform passive stretching exercises, the torticollis will resolve. Remnants of the third and fourth branchial arches and clefts may be found as cysts, pits, or tracks. Usually these do not require excision and can be observed. Another type of cyst, which also may be found in the neck, is a cystic hygroma. These cysts originate from the lymphatic system and sometimes occur in the axilla and groin. Midline lesions in the neck are more often associated with the thyroglossal duct and the thyroid gland. Webbing of the neck may occur, most prominently in Turner's syndrome (XO chromosomes).

The shape and size of the bony *thorax* should be noted and the clavicles palpated to make sure that they were not fractured during the birthing process. Sometimes the practitioner is alerted to a clavicular fracture, because the infant is not moving one of its arms or the infant has an asymmetrical Moro reflex (described later).

The *chest* examination may reveal breast buds or gynecomastia that result from exposure to the maternal hormones. Sometimes milk can be expressed from these infant buds, and rarely, mastitis may occur. Nipples that are widely spaced or an abnormally shaped chest would alert the pediatrician to look for other abnormalities associated with congenital syndromes. From time to time, supernumerary nipples will be present. They can occur at any point on the nipple line, which runs from the axilla to the groin. They are of no particular clinical significance.

Asymmetry or an abnormal contour of the *abdomen* alerts the examiner to the possibility of a mass or diaphragmatic hernia. All four quadrants of the infant's abdomen must be felt for masses, and then the liver, spleen, and kidneys must be palpated individually. In most newborns, it is possible to feel the right kidney easily, and very often with bimanual palpation and ballotment, the left can also be felt. The liver edge is usually felt at 1 to 2 cm below the right costal margin, but the spleen should not be palpable.

Careful examination of the *anus* should make sure that it is in the normal position and is distally patent. A complete ring of stria around the anus reassures the examiner that the "anus" is not actually a fistula.

The *spine* should be palpated to make sure that there are no defects or dimples. Pits or hair tufts raise the possibility of abnormality and require further evaluation, such as an ultrasound of the spine.

In examining the *male genitalia*, a small scrotal sac may indicate that the testes are undescended, and asymmetry may indicate the presence of a hydrocele, a hernia, or the unilateral absence of a testis. The normal range of penile length is 2.5 to 4.5 cm, measured from the pubic bone to the tips of the glans. The urethral meatus should be slit-like and positioned at the tip of the glans. If the meatus is displaced, the infant should not be circumcised. Management of hypospadias depends on its degree and should be done in consultation with a pediatric urologist.

On observation of the *female genitalia*, the labia, the clitoris, and the introitus should be within the normal range of variation. The labia majora should be as big as, or bigger than, the labia minora. It is normal to see a white mucous discharge and even withdrawal bleeding from the maternal estrogens in female infants. Another common finding is a pink, fleshy looking vaginal skin tag. This tag will reabsorb by itself.

If there is any question of *ambiguous genitalia*, a full evaluation should be done so that the most appropriate sex can be assigned to the infant. Once a sex has been assigned to an infant, it is psychologically and emotionally disruptive to parents and family to change the assignation.

Carefully examine *hips* to make sure that they are not dislocated or dislocatable. The Ortolani and Barlow maneuvers are used; see Table 16.4.

Body symmetry is important, as is *proportionality*. The length of the baby should always be greater than the span (measured from middle finger tip to middle finger tip with the arms outstretched). Legs should be longer than arms. When arms hang at the side, they should reach down to midthigh.

Fingers and *toes* should be counted. It is not uncommon to find either supernumerary digits or syndactyly, as they are both dominant traits that run in families. If the family wishes, supernumerary digits can be removed and syndactyly can be separated. Examine the feet

Table 16.4   Ortalani's and Barlow's tests (each test is one figure)

Hips are flexed to 90 degrees and instability is detected by:
- Reduction of dislocation by abduction and forward pressure (Ortalani's test)
- Dislocation of hip by adduction and backward pressure (Barlow's test)

to make sure that there is no talipes equino varus (clubfoot) or other nonpositional abnormalities that require orthopedic evaluation.

It is most important to evaluate the *muscle tone*, the presence and symmetry of the primitive reflexes and the deep tendon reflexes. Low tone is always abnormal; the examiner should immediately review the history and look for other signs and symptoms to find a cause. The low tone may be a manifestation of trisomy 21 (Down syndrome) or it may merely reflect a high magnesium level due to the mother receiving magnesium sulfate to treat preeclampsia. High tone may be seen in infants undergoing withdrawal from maternal narcotics, and generally, this condition will appear in the hours or days following delivery. Some infants seem to be very jittery, and, although it may be a normal variant, it is important to ascertain that the infant is not hypoglycemic, hypocalcemic, hypomagnesemic, or undergoing neonatal abstinence syndrome.

The Moro or startle reflex is elicited by dropping the infant's head backward into the examiner's hand, at the same time supporting the body with the examiner's arms. Normal infants respond by symmetrically abducting the arms and extending the fingers, followed by a return to the flexed posture. Asymmetry of the Moro may be the clue to a fractured clavicle or an Erb's palsy. An Erb's palsy involves varying amount of injury to the fifth and sixth cervical nerves as they pass through the brachial plexus. The much rarer Klumpke's palsy involves the seventh and eighth cervical and first thoracic nerves. Both are usually a result of a difficult delivery where the shoulders are wider than the presenting part (the head) and the nerve roots are stretched or, rarely, avulsed.

The *skin* of term newborns may still have remnants of the cheesy material called vernix caseosa, which consists of sebum and desquamated epithelial cells, but most of the downy fetal hair will have been shed. You may see some minor peeling of the skin. Severe cracking and dryness of the skin indicates a postdate or postmature infant. You may also note that a postmature infant has a decreased amount of subcutaneous tissue and looks somewhat scrawny compared to the plump look of a term infant. Some newborns have a very ruddy skin color, which may be an indication of polycythemia. Most of the time, polycythemia has no negative consequences per se; however, it means that the infant has a higher red cell load to break down, which may lead to a higher level of bilirubin and clinical jaundice. Polycythemia, especially at a high altitude, may be associated with hyperviscosity syndrome. Any hematocrit over 60 should be rechecked and any over 65 from a central stick should be treated (see Appendix A).

Newborns may have several minor evanescent rashes that are benign and require no treatment. However, some skin rashes may be a cause of great concern for the parents and at times need to be distinguished from more serious skin eruptions by the pediatrician. The following is a list of the most common:

- Superficial epidermal inclusion cysts may appear on the facial skin as milia or be found on the hard palate as Epstein's pearls or the gums as Bohn's nodules.

- Sebaceous hyperplasia is common and causes minute yellow-white papules on the forehead, nose, cheeks, and upper lip of newborns.

- Erythema toxicum and transient neonatal pustular melanosis are two benign rashes whose lesions might be confused with herpes simplex lesions or staphylococcal pustules. Usually their distinctive morphology enables differentiation, but if a gram stain and Tzanck preparation of the lesions is done, erythema toxicum lesions will show eosinophils on gram stain, staphylococcal lesions will show bacteria on gram stain, and herpetic lesions will show giant cells on Tzanck prep. Culture of the lesions will also provide more information, but will take 48 to 72 hours.

- Salmon patches (nevus flammeus, stork's bite, or angels' kisses) are capillary hemangiomas that are commonly found at the nape of the neck and on the eyelids, glabella, and upper lip. The lesions fade over time, although the stork bite mark at the nape of the neck may persist into adulthood. Parents often report that they can tell when their child is angry or unwell (or both), as they can see the faint mark of the hemangioma return!

- Mongolian spots are bluish/black areas found most frequently in the sacral area, but also may occur anywhere on the body. They are due to the presence of spindle-shaped pigment cells deep in the dermis. They are more common in infants who generally have more pigment, and they tend to fade with time, although they may persist into adult life.

SUGGESTED READING

Surgical-tutor.org.uk. <www.surgical-tutor.org.uk.> 01 Jan 2001.
Neonatology on the Web. <http://www.neonatology.org/ref/dubowitz.html.> 28 Nov 1995.

CHAPTER 17

Newborn and Infant Growth and Development Charts

Gary A. Emmett

Some convenient charts for judging a newborn's development and growth percentiles.

The following are three helpful sets of charts:

- An adaptation of the Ballard/Dubowitz gestational developmental tables with explanations

- The new growth and development charts for children from birth to age 3 years from the centers for Disease Control and Prevention (CDC)

- A modification of gestational age versus size chart based on Babson and Benda

Epidermal inclusion cysts

gums ↓ Bohn's nodules

hard palate ↓ Epstein pearls

Table 17.1 Neuromuscular maturity from Ballard/Dubowitz chart

Directions for scoring: Score all measures with infant supine and quiet.

Posture: See chart.

Square window: Flex the hand at the wrist until resistance occurs. Measure the angle from the anterior aspect of the forearm to the base of the thumb (hypothenar eminence).

Arm recoil: Fully flex the forearms for 5 sec, then fully extend by pulling the hands and release. Measure the angle at the elbow.

Popliteal angle: Score with pelvis flat on the examining surface. Fully flex the thigh with one hand. With the other hand, extend the leg until resistance occurs. Measure the posterior angle.

Scarf sign: Take the infant's hand and draw it across the neck to the opposite shoulder until resistance occurs. If the chest obstructs elbow, the elbow may be lifted across the body. Note location of the elbow.

Heel to ear: Score with pelvis flat on the examining surface. Hold the infant's foot with one hand and move it toward the head until resistance occurs. Measure posterior angle of the knee.

Total Score on Ballard-Dubowitz	Gestational age in weeks
5	26
10	28
15	30
20	32
25	34
30	36
35	38
40	40
45	42
50	44

Sign/Score	−1	0	1	2	3	4	5	Scoring
Posture		Arms and legs extended	Slight flexion of hips/ knees	Moderate/ strong flexion of hips/knees	Legs flexed, arms slightly flexed	Full flexion arms/legs		
Square window (degrees)	>90	90	60	45	30	0		
Arm recoil (degrees)		Remains extended (180)	Minimal flexion (140–180)	Small flexion (110–140)	Moderate flexion (90–100)	Full flexion (<90)		
Popliteal angle (degrees)	180	160	140	120	100	90	<90	
Scarf sign	Elbow on or near opposite shoulder	Elbow crosses opposite anterior axillary line	Elbow reaches opposite anterior axillary line	Elbow at midline	Elbow does not reach midline	Elbow does not cross proximate axillary line		
Heel to ear (degrees)	171–180	151–170	121–150	91–120	90	<90		

Total neuromuscular maturity score _____

TABLE 17.2 Physical maturity from Ballard/Dubowitz chart

Sign/Score	-1	0	1	2	3	4	5	Scoring
Skin	Sticky, friable, transparent	Gelatinous, red, translucent	Smooth, pink, visible veins	Superficial peeling and/or rash, few veins	Cracking, pale areas, rare veins	Parchment, deep cracking, no vessels	Leathery, cracked, wrinkled	
Lanugo	None	Sparse	Abundant	Thinning	Bald areas	Mostly bald		
Plantar creases	Heel to toe 40–50 mm	Heel to toe >50 mm, no creases	Faint red marks	Anterior transverse crease only	Deep creases over anterior 2/3	Deep creases over entire sole		
Breast	Imperceptible	Barely perceptible	Flat areola, no bud	Stippled areola, 1–2 mm bud	Raised areola, 3–4 mm bud	Full areola, 5–10 mm bud		
Eye and ear	Lids fused loosely	Lids open and pinna flat, ear stays folded	Slightly curved pinna, soft with slow recoil	Well-curved pinna, soft but ready recoil	Ear formed/firm, with instant recoil	Thick cartilage, ear stiff		
Genitals (male)	Scrotum flat, smooth	Scrotum empty, faint rugae	Testes in upper canal, rare rugae	Testes descending, few rugae	Testes descended, defined rugae	Testes pendulous, deep rugae		
Genitals (female)	Clitoris prominent, labia flat	Prominent clitoris, small labia minora	Prominent clitoris, enlarging minora	Labia majora = minora	Labia majora > minora	Labia majora covers clitoris/ minora		

Total physical maturity score _____

Total score (add neuromuscular and physical scores) _____

TABLE 17.3   Gestational age from Ballard/Dubowitz scoring

Use the Total Score of the Ballard/Dubowitz charts (Tables 17.1 and 17.2) to determine gestational age.

Total Score	−10	−5	0	5	10	15	20	25	30	35	40	45	50
Gestational Age, Weeks	20	22	24	26	28	30	32	34	36	38	40	42	44

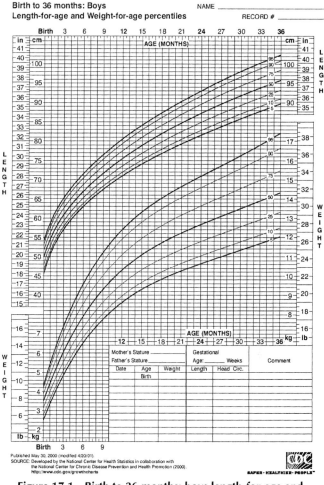

Figure 17.1   Birth to 36 months: boys length-for-age and weight-for-age percentiles.

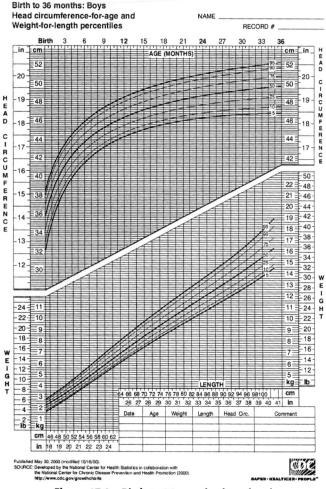

Figure 17.2   Birth to 36 months: boys head circumference-for-age and weight-for-length percentiles.

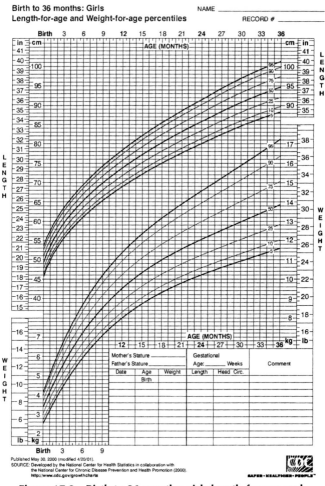

Figure 17.3   Birth to 36 months: girls length-for-age and weight-for-age percentiles.

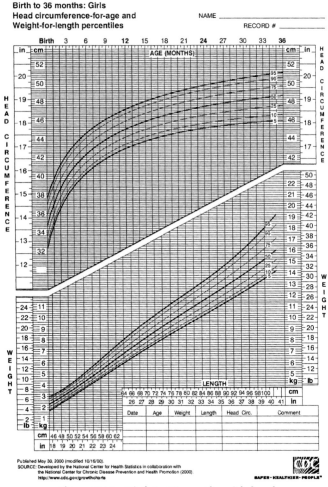

Figure 17.4 Birth to 36 months: girls head circumference-for-age and weight-for-length percentiles.

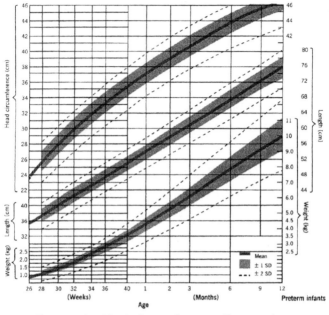

Figure 17.5   Physical growth percentiles at various gestational ages.

SUGGESTED READING

Advance Data. <www.cdc.gov/nchs/data/ad/ad314.pdf> 16 Nov 2000.

Ballard JL, Novak KK, Driver M. A simplified score for assessment of fetal maturation of newly born infants, *J Pediatr* 1979;95:709–774.

BabyCenter.com Growth Percentile Calculator. <www.babycenter.com/growthchart/> Dec 2003.

Babson SG, Benda GI. Growth graphs for the clinical assessment of infants of varying gestational age. *J Pediatr* 1976;89:815.

Ballard JL, Khovry JC, Wedig K, Wang L, Eilers-Walsman BL, Lippu R. New Ballard Score, expanded to include extremely premature infants. *J Pediatr* 1991;119:417–423.

CHAPTER 18

Teratogens: Prenatal Maternal Drugs Producing Congenital Defects

Gary A. Emmett

Almost no medications in the United States are listed as being safe during pregnancy, because the market is too small to justify the cost of testing them in pregnant women.

This chapter is simply two tables: a long list of drugs that are currently thought to produce birth defects if taken during pregnancy and a list of drugs formerly thought to be dangerous, but now deemed safe. A caveat: Only 2% to 3% of congenital defects are secondary to medication. The list is very complete for antiepileptic medications, because they are so commonly used in pregnancy. Neuroactive drugs that produce withdrawal are listed in Chapter 19.

Table 18.1   Teratogens and their effects

Teratogen	Material Problem	Trimester of Effect	Most Common Effects
Ace inhibitors	Hypertension	2nd and 3rd	Renal effects: neonatal renal failure, oligohydramnios, pulmonary hypoplasia
Aminopterin, methotrexate, and other similar antimetabolites	Cancer	1st (3–10 wk)	Skull, eye, and skeletal defects with large fontanelles
Antithyroid agents	Hyperthyroidism	End of 1st, 2nd, 3rd	Neonate hypothyroidism, goiter
Anticholinergic drugs	Increased secretions	3rd	Meconium ileus
Carbamazepine	Epilepsy	1st (3–10 wk)	Neural tube defects
Clonazepam	Epilepsy	1st (3–10 wk)	Not clear, almost always taken with other antiepleptics
Cocaine	Drug of abuse	1st and 2nd	Arterial spasm with regional ischemia
Coumarin/warfarin	Clots	Late 1st	Nasal hypoplasia and other CNS/facial defects
Cyclophosphamide	Transplanted organ	1st (3–10 wk)	Skeletal defects, cleft palate
Ethanol	Drug of abuse, solvent	1st and 2nd	Fetal alcohol syndrome
Danazol	Endometriosis, hereditary angioedema	All	Virilization of females
Diethylstilbestrol	Ovarian insufficiency, postcoital contraception	1st, 2nd	Vaginal/cervical carcinoma as young adults
Fluconazole	Fungus	1st	Syndrome of skull defects, heart disease, arthrogryposis, multiple bone thinning and bowing

(continued)

Table 18.1 (Continued)

Teratogen	Material Problem	Trimester of Effect	Most Common Effects
Hypoglycemic drugs	Diabetes	3rd	Neonatal hypoglycemia
Indomethacin	Nonsteroidal antiinflammatory agent	2nd, 3rd	Oligohydramnios, early closure of PDA, NEC
Isotretinoin and other retinoids	Severe acne	1st (3–10 wk)	Retinoid embryopathy*
Lithium	Manic-depressive disorder	1st (3–10 wk)	Ebstein's anomaly, tricuspid defects
Methimazole	Hyperthyroidism	All	Hyperthyroidism; scalp, skull, nail, and nipple defects; atresia of choanus and esophagus
Methylene blue	Amniocentesis	2nd	Jejunal atresia
Misoprostol	Ulcers, abortions	1st, beginning of 2nd	Moebius anomaly, distal limb aplasia, arthrogryposis
Phenobarbital	Epilepsy	1st (3–10 wk)	Facial clefting, heart disease, nail hypoplasia
Phenytoin	Antiseizure	1st, beginning 2nd	Cleft palate, micromelia, hydrocephalus
Primidone	Antiepileptic	1st (3–10 wk)	Similar to phenobarbital, but also hirsute forehead
Tetracycline	Infection, acne	2nd, 3rd	Dental staining and weakening
Thalidomide	Insomnia, immune disease	27–40 days	Limb reduction, multiorgan defects
Trimethoprim	Infection	1st	Neural tube defects, oral clefts, hypospadias, heart disease
Valproic acid	Epilepsy, mental disease	1st	Neural tube defects

*Hydrocephalus, ear defects, micrognathia, cleft lip/palate, tetralogy of Fallot and other defects of heart and great vessels, face defects, eye defects, limb hypoplasia and aplasia, and others. Women on Accutane and other retinoids must be checked for pregnancy before and during use.

Table 18.2 Drugs formerly thought to be teratogens and now deemed safe

- Bendectin (Diclectin)
- Diazepam
- Oral contraceptives
- Spermicides
- Aspirin and other salicylates

SUGGESTED READING

Polifka JE, Friedman JM. Medical genetics: 1. Clinical teratology in the age of genomics. *Can Med Assoc J* 2002;167:265–273.

Finnell RH. Teratology: general considerations and principles. *J Allergy Clin Immunol* 1999;103:S337–42.

Koren G, Pastuszak A, Ito S. Drugs in pregnancy. *New Engl J Med* 1998;228:1128–1137.

CHAPTER 19

Effects of Maternal Drug Use in Newborns

Gary A. Emmett

We know what neuroactive substances do to newborns immediately after birth, but the controversial question is, what do they do to the child in kindergarten?

When a pregnant woman takes a neuroactive substance, the substance also affects her fetus. Fetuses are affected by legal compounds (caffeine, ethanol, glucose, and nicotine) and banned substances (amphetamines, barbiturates, benzodiazepams, cocaine, opiates, and derivatives PCP and THC). This chapter details the effects of these substances on newborn behavior and describes neonatal abstinence syndrome. Exposure to neuroactive substances in utero can be long-term and devastating. Sudden infant death is strongly associated with babies whose mothers smoked or used alcohol during pregnancy; it is increased in those who were exposed to cocaine and amphetamines prenatally. In addition, alcohol and cocaine exposure often have long-term intellectual damage that is never corrected.

If a mother is known or suspected of taking neuroactive substances, a urine screen in the mother and the baby for drugs of abuse is recommended. Mothers who have had very poor prenatal care or have a history of losing their children to social welfare agencies should also be checked regularly for drugs of abuse. In all cases of infant exposure to neuroactive substances in utero, the social work department of the hospital should be involved.

The effects of neuroactive substances in newborns are nearly identical to the effects in adults. The withdrawals are also remarkably similar to those of adults, except that newborns are much more prone toward apnea than adults. Those substances, such as barbiturates and benzodiazepams, that can suppress breathing suppress it even more significantly in newborns. The effects and withdrawal symptoms of various substances are described in Table 19.1.

Pregnant women frequently ingest *caffeine*. Caffeine and other theobromides are found in coffee, tea, many soda pops, chocolate, and many common over-the-counter medications such as no-doze and diet pills. Babies who are born with a high level of caffeine in their system are hypervigilant and have hyperreflexia. Withdrawal in the newborn often does not occur, because the breast-feeding mother continues to supply the theobromide compounds she ingested during pregnancy. If a mother decides to stop taking caffeine, the baby's supply is cut off quickly, and the baby will be very irritable and unable to settle. Caffeine withdrawal

Table 19.1   Short-term effects of neuroactive substances used by mother during pregnancy

	Postpartum effects	Withdrawal
Licit		
Caffeine	High activity level, poor sleeping	Extreme irritability, high-pitched cry
Ethanol	Fetal alcohol syndrome, hepatitis, microcephaly	High-pitched cry, irritability, seizure
Glucose	Microsomia, heart defects	Hypoglycemia, seizures
Nicotine	Increased wakefulness, dry mouth, small pupils	Irritability, high-pitched cry
Illicit		
Amphetamines	Extreme irritability, brain damage	No classic withdrawal
Barbiturates	Somnolence	Extreme irritability, apnea
Benzodiazepams	Somnolence	Extreme irritability, apnea
Cocaine	Prolonged irritability and agitation	None, but possible permanent brain damage
Opiates	Somnolence	Irritability, clonus, loose stools (see Table 19.3)
PCP and THC	Somnolence	PCP, unknown; THC, no withdrawal, but sedation may be prolonged

in newborns is usually a short-term phenomenon and is gone in 2 to 3 days. Serious side effects are extremely rare.

Caffeine is often used medically in apneic babies to encourage spontaneous breathing, but in that situation withdrawal is rare, because the babies are usually allowed to grow out of their medication. Theophylline is still used in asthma treatment, though it is rare at the beginning of the 21st century. Sudden cessation of theophylline will have an effect similar to that of sudden withdrawal of caffeine.

Ethanol, drinking alcohol, is the most common drug of abuse in the world. Although alcohol abuse can cause many problems in the newborn, primarily intrauterine growth retardation, microcephaly, fatty hepatitis, and even feminization of males, the most serious problem

Table 19.2   Signs and symptoms of fetal alcohol syndrome

- Macrosomia/microcephaly
- Unusual eye folds
- Small maxilla
- Flat, wide philtrum
- Delayed development
- ADHD-like syndrome

from alcohol is fetal alcohol syndrome. Fetal alcohol syndrome is more common with increasing maternal alcohol ingestion, but may occur in mothers who drank only sporadically during pregnancy. The irregular pattern found implies that both environmental toxicity and host susceptibility are involved. Fetal alcohol syndrome is difficult to recognize immediately after birth and is usually not picked up until the developmental delay and hyperactivity become evident. The clarity of the peculiar facial features becomes obvious only when the physician looks for a cause of the neurological problems. Withdrawal is very rare in babies exposed to high levels of alcohol. Table 19.2 lists the signs and symptoms of fetal alcohol syndrome.

Glucose is a problem mainly in the subsequent production of high levels of insulin in the newborn (see Chapters 7 and 21).

Up to 25% of pregnant women smoke *cigarettes* during their pregnancy. Nicotine causes fetal growth retardation in babies whose mothers smoke a pack of cigarettes a day or more; these babies weigh on the average 200 grams less than babies whose mothers do not smoke. Nicotine's symptoms and withdrawal are usually mitigated by the mother's continued use of tobacco. Breast-feeding mothers will easily transfer nicotine to the baby, and even smoking in the same room usually transfers enough nicotine to prevent severe withdrawal. Problems arise primarily when the baby is separated from the mother, usually because one or the other is ill. Nicotine reduces the need for sleep and in large doses can cause high activity levels in users. Withdrawal is primarily irritability and has not been known to be severe and certainly not fatal.

Amphetamines are associated with premature delivery and growth retardation in utero. Amphetamines also cause decreased appetite and decreased food intake in the mother. Separating the effects of poor diet from the direct effects of the drug is difficult, and therefore, the intrauterine growth retardation may be associated with maternal diet and not amphetamines. Amphetamines, in general, are very short-lived, so the effects of amphetamine withdrawal are much more likely to be observed than amphetamine toxicity. Babies whose mothers have taken significant doses of amphetamines have irritability, a shrill cry, sneezing, sweating, intermittent drowsiness, and increased myoclonic jerks.

Treatment of this irritability usually consists of "papoosing" (wrapping the baby firmly in its blankets), feeding, and gentle rhythmic motion.

Barbiturates and *benzodiazepams* are associated with initial somnolence and poor muscle tone in exposed neonates. They are both associated with interuterine growth retardation and with poor maternal diets. They can cause apnea, either from toxicity or in withdrawal. Some of them have extremely long half-lives in the child and may produce withdrawal up to a week after the baby is born. Infants exposed to these medications should be watched for at least 72 hours in the hospital in a monitored bed. In extreme cases, with very long acting substances, treatment may be needed for withdrawal symptoms.

Cocaine is a stimulant that blocks the reuptake of catecholamines at nerve terminals. Along with producing intoxication, cocaine may produce vasospasm. Arterial vasospasm in utero may produce ischemia and loss of segments of bowel or brain. Cocaine babies are very small, because people on high doses of cocaine do not eat. The effects of cocaine in the newborn are numerous. The rate of stillbirths and prematurity in cocaine users is high. After birth, babies are extremely irritable, and their Brazelton developmental scores are abnormal until at least the second birthday. These children are probably permanently abnormally developed, but the only controlled long-term study has shown that poor home environments obscure the effects of the cocaine by the time the child enters kindergarten. Cocaine is very short acting and does not appear to have a classic withdrawal syndrome.

Heroin and methadone are the most commonly encountered *opiates* in the newborn nursery. Heroin is very short acting, and withdrawal is usually within 6 hours. Methadone is very long acting and can stay in the baby's system for many days. Withdrawal has occurred as late as 2 to 3 weeks in the newborn from exposure to methadone. Initially, opiates produce somnolence and occasional apnea. The withdrawal from opiates has a classic set of central nervous system, metabolic, respiratory, and gastrointestinal presentations. The commonly used device to allow quantification of infant withdrawal may be a modification of Dr. Lauretta Finnegan's neonatal abstinence score. The version used at Thomas Jefferson University Hospital, Philadelphia, Pennsylvania, is found in Table 19.3.

The treatment of opiate withdrawal has no uniform pattern in the United States. Because heroin withdrawal, although associated with great discomfort, is not fatal, some do not treat neonatal abstinence syndrome with medications. These practitioners use papoosing, sucking, rhythmic motion, and human contact to take the babies through this lengthy process. We cannot recommend this approach. Multiple drugs have been used, including benzodiazepams, barbiturates, and opiates. Currently, the use of a water suspension of opium is one recommendation. For alternative medication, see Table 19.4.

Table 19.3 Neonatal abstinence scoring

Scoring should be done before each feeding. Scoring is operator dependent and improves with experience. Three scores totaling 24 may indicate that treatment is needed.

Date	Weight	Score	AM	PM	Comments
System	Signs and symptoms				
CNS disturbances	Excessive high-pitched cry *or*	2			
	continuous high-pitched cry	3			
	Sleeps <1 hr after feeding *or*	3			
	Sleeps <2 hr after feeding *or*	2			
	Sleeps <3 hr after feeding	1			
	Hyperactive MORO reflex *or*	2			
	Markedly hyperactive MORO reflex	3			
	Mild tremors disturbed *or*	1			
	Moderate–severe tremors disturbed	2			
	Mild tremors undisturbed *or*	3			
	Moderate–severe tremors undisturbed	4			
	Increased muscle tone	2			
	Excoriation (esp. diaper area)	1			
	Myoclonic jerks	3			
	Generalized convulsions	5			

Metabolic, nasal, respiratory disturbances	Sweating	1
	Fever <101 (99–100°F/37.2–38.2°C) *or*	1
	Fever >101 (38.4°C and higher)	2
	Frequent yawning (>3–4 times/interval)	1
	Mottling	1
	Nasal stuffiness	1
	Sneezing (>3–4 times/interval)	1
	Nasal flaring	2
	Respiratory rate >60/min *or*	1
	Resp. rate >60/min with retractions	2
GI disturbances	Excessive sucking	1
	Poor feeding	2
	Regurgitation *or*	2
	projectile vomiting	3
	Loose stools *or*	2
	watery stools	3
	Total score:	
	Scorers initials	

Table 19.4   Treatment of opiate withdrawal

Opium water suspension (standard tincture of opium 1 cc added to 24 mL sterile water, which is equal to 0.4 mg morphine sulfate, MSO_4, per cc)

- Starting dose: 0.4 mg MSO_4 per 24 hr, divided into equal doses, before each feeding.
- Increase by 0.04 mg/kg/day (0.1 cc), divided into equal doses, prior to feeding until control is achieved.
- Control is demonstrated by average neonatal abstinence score of less than 8, regular feeding/sleep cycles, and weight gain of 15 g per day or more.
- If stable for 72 hr, decrease 10% every 24–48 hr as long as child remains in control.

Phenobarbital
- 15–20 mg/kg loading dose IM or PO.
- Followed by 4–6 mg/kg/day maintenance given BID.
- Paragoric may be added to the four drops orally every 4 hr as needed for control (see above).
- If stable for 72 hr, decrease 10% every 24–48 hr as long as child remains in control.

Nonmedicinal
- Papoosing
- Rhythmic motion
- Frequent feeding
- Human contact

PCP (phencyclidine or angel dust) has limited experience noted in neonates. In the few case reports available, it is clear that PCP rapidly crosses the placenta and may cause poor feeding, increased tone, and irritability in newborns. Long-term effects are unknown. Frank withdrawal has not been noted.

As many as 16% of all mothers smoke or ingest *THC* (tetrahydrocannabinol) during their pregnancy, most commonly by smoking marijuana. Reports of its effects on the newborn are numerous but completely contradictory. Partially, this is because THC is often ingested with other neuroactive substances. Withdrawal does not seem to be an issue, but because THC is small and highly fat soluble, fetuses can have brain levels higher than their mothers.

Most other frequently used substances, such as Ecstasy (MDMA) and LSD, have no generally acknowledged effect because of minimal reports.

SUGGESTED READING

Literature citations site of the National Council of Biotech Information. <http://www.ncbi.nlm.nih.gov/entrez/query.fcgi>

Belik J, Al-Hamad N. Neonatal abstinence syndrome. *eMed J.* <http://author.emedicine.com/ped/topic2760.htm> May 2003.

CHAPTER 20
Breast-feeding When Mothers Are Taking Prescribed Medication

Gary A. Emmett

With breast-feeding, everything that the mother eats ends up to some extent in the baby. Most substances that are not harming the mother are not harming the baby.

Table 20.1 provides guidelines from the American Academy of Pediatrics (AAP) regarding drug therapy for lactating women. Very few circumstances prohibit breast-feeding completely. Mothers who are positive for HIV should not breast-feed, but only if bottle-feeding will not lead to malnutrition or disease (see Chapter 12). Some sources suggest that breast-feeding is forbidden while the mother is on antimetabolites, warfarin, or tricyclic antidepressants, but in real life, many babies have successfully breast-fed on all three. Table 20.2 consists of lists that suggest that certain medications are not encouraged while a mother is breast-feeding, but nothing in this chapter is absolute, because there are no controlled data to back up the lists. Some maternal medications have only one case report of subsequent problems in the newborn. Appendix C is a more complete list of the effects of maternal use of medications on breast-feeding babies.

Table 20.1 AAP rules for drug therapy of the lactating woman

1. Is the drug really necessary?
2. Use the safest drug (acetaminophen, not aspirin, for example).
3. If there is concern about the drug level in the nursing child, check the blood level.
4. Drugs are best given just after breast-feeding and just before the child has a long sleep period.

Table 20.2   Ingested substances that may cause problems in breast-feeding

Antimetabolites

Cyclophosphamide, cyclosporine, doxorubicin, methotrexate	May cause immune suppression, poor growth, neutropenia

Drugs of abuse

Alcohol	With large amounts: somnolence, sweating, poor growth, fatty liver, feminization
Amphetamine	Poor sleep cycle, irritability
Cocaine	Diarrhea and vomiting, seizures
Heroin	Vomiting, poor intake, somnolence
Marijuana	Somnolence
PCP	Hallucinations

Environmental and food substances in breast milk that may harm the newborn

Aspartame	Brain damage if child has PKU
Bromide	Teeth staining, weakness, no cry
Caffeine	If high dosage, irritability, erratic sleep cycle
Chocolate, coffee	Irritability
Fava beans	Hemolysis if child has G-6-PD
Heavy metals	May decrease developmental potential
Poly-chlorinated (-brominated) biphenyls	Poor tone, "frozen" face
Strict vegan diet	Macrocytic anemia secondary to B_{12} deficiency

Medications associated with multiple reports of side effects in nursing children

Acebutolol	Hypotension, bradycardia
Atenolol	Cyanosis, bradycardia
Bromocriptine	Dehydration (reduces mother's lactation)
Carbimazole	Goiter
Ergotamine	Vomiting, diarrhea, symptoms of ergotism
Lithium	Blood levels up to 1/2 of mother's
Phenobarbital	Sedation
SSRIs (i.e., Prozac)	Colic, irritability, poor feeding/weight gain
Sulfa drugs	If child has G-6-PD and jaundice, can worsen

(continued)

Table 20.2   (*Continued*)

Radioactive substances
May cause significant radiation in infant. Pump and store breast milk before procedure and avoid substances such as gallium 67 with very long 1/2 lives (in the case of gallium 67 detectable for over 2 wk in breast milk).

SUGGESTED READING

American Academy of Pediatrics Committee on Drugs. Transfer of drugs and other chemicals into human milk, a review with 392 references. *Pediatrics* 2001;108:776–789.

CHAPTER 21

Maternal Disease Producing Neonatal Problems

Gary A. Emmett

Sometimes childhood disease is only a reflection of the mother's health.

Many diseases in childhood are only reflections of maternal disease. The two most common examples are neonatal hypoglycemia secondary to maternal diabetes (see Chapters 7 and 22) and hemolytic disease of the newborn secondary to maternal blood group antibodies (see Chapter 15). Table 21.1 is an alphabetical list of symptoms and signs found in the newborn and the maternal conditions that the practitioner should investigate and possibly ameliorate.

Table 21.1   Neonatal illness secondary to maternal disease

Symptom/Sign	Maternal Condition
Erythema of face, photosensitive	Lupus
Heart block	Lupus
Hemolysis of newborn	Blood group incompatibility. Mother with the null genotype for an erythrocyte blood group: $(-)$ in Rh, O in ABO, O in MNO, $(-)$ in Lewis, Kell, or Duffy; while child is $(+)$: $(+)$ in Rh, Lewis, Kell, or Duffy or MNO, A, or B in ABO.
Hydrops fetalis	• Lupus • Blood group incompatibility
Hyperviscosity/ polycythemia	• Hypoxia • Cigarette smoking • Living at high altitude
Hypoglycemia	Hyperglycemia/diabetes
Macrosomia	Hyperglycemia/diabetes
Neural tube defect/ spina bifida	Folate deficiency (although folate is now in every product containing flour, advise the mother of a child with a neural tube defect to take 1 mg of folate daily)
Ptosis	• Myasthenia gravis • Botulism

CHAPTER 22

Large and Small Babies

Gary A. Emmett

Always consider the parental size before worrying about the child's size.

To determine if a newborn is abnormally large or small, refer to Fig.17.5. To classify a baby as large or small for gestational age, the newborn must be more than two standard deviations from the mean as shown on this chart. As of April 2004, the CDC has not released new data on newborn size, but information may be released soon.

Always consider the child's size in the context of parental size and prenatal history before doing a major workup. In general, tall people have tall and therefore large babies, and short people have short and therefore small babies. Studies have shown that the maternal size is the more important contributor for the newborn. Tanner has shown that both parents contribute to eventual height, with the same-sex parent contributing about twice as much influence as the opposite-sex parent.

If a full-term newborn baby's weight is 5 kg (11 lb and greater than the 95th percentile) and its length is 48.5 cm (19 in. and 40th percentile), consider hyperinsulinemia secondary to maternal diabetes and treat the child very aggressively. But, if an infant of the same weight is 55 cm long (21.7 in. and greater than the 95th percentile), the chance of initial hypoglycemia is much less. It is likely that this newborn is the product of large parents and may not have been exposed to high glucose levels in utero. Likewise, a baby born to a 40-kg (88 lb.), 147-cm (58 in.) mother is not necessarily abnormal if it weighs 2 kg (4 lb, 7 oz) and has a proportional length.

All *large for gestational age* (LGA) babies should have their serum glucose followed for the first 4 to 8 hours of life. Although it is normal for large parents to give birth to LGA babies, a large mother may have elevated serum glucose during pregnancy, and, in fact, if she is obese, the chances of maternal hyperglycemia are higher than average. Even if the baby is LGA and of proportional length for weight to the parents, the baby's serum glucose levels must be followed. Table 22.1 lists causes of LGA infants.

Table 22.2 lists causes of newborn hyperinsulinemia. If the mother has type I diabetes (juvenile), then there are two opposing forces that determine a child's size:

1. The tendency of glucose crossing the placenta to induce increased fetal insulin and somatomedin production. The production of both, in turn, induces increased in utero growth

2. The tendency of long-standing diabetics to have vasculitis of the small vessels, decreasing the blood flow to the fetus and thus decreasing the infant's size (see later section on small infants)

Table 22.1   Primary causes of large for gestational age (LGA) infants

- Large maternal size (primarily height)
- Hyperinsulinemia, usually caused by maternal hyperglycemia
- Congenital overgrowth syndromes with multiple congenital defects (rare)

The most common cause of high glucose exposure in infancy is gestational diabetes. Gestational diabetes is usually seen in mothers with a family history of type II diabetes (adult onset). These mothers rarely have any vascular problems, so these babies can become very large if the mother's hyperglycemia is untreated.

Rarely, a child is LGA and has profound hypoglycemia of the newborn that does not respond to glucose. Even if the intravenous glucose does raise the child's blood sugar, the euglycemia will disappear as soon as the intravenous is removed, and the glucose can plunge to zero almost instantly. In these cases, seizures commonly occur. These children may have a tumor such as a nesidioblastoma or insulinoma of the pancreas.

Although extremely rare (less than one in 10,000 births), some LGA babies have congenital overgrowth syndromes. Beckwith-Wiedemann and the closely related syndrome of hemihypertrophy are the most common of the congenital overgrowth syndromes with multiple congenital defects. Beckwith-Wiedemann children have large tongues, are of large size (macrosomic), have organomegaly (large liver and spleen), and occasionally, have an omphalocele (lack of closure of the abdominal cavity). They also have peculiar horizontal creases on their earlobes. A single gene defect on chromosome 11 is known to be causative, and the presentation is sporadic. There is at least a 6.5% chance of children with Beckwith-Wiedemann developing a malignant tumor during early childhood. These children have profound and long-lasting hypoglycemia and are often brain-damaged if diagnosis and treatment of the low serum glucose is delayed.

Hemihypertrophy syndrome is a different defect at the same locus on chromosome 11 as Beckwith-Wiedemann. In addition to the symptoms just listed, babies with hemihypertrophy have a peculiar presentation where one half of the body, usually the left, is of normal size and one

Table 22.2   Causes of newborn hyperinsulinemia

- Maternal type I diabetes (infant may or may not be large)
- Maternal type II diabetes
- Infant insulin-producing tumor

Table 22.3   Syndromes of congenital macrosomia with multiple congenital defects

Disease	Symptoms/Signs
Beckwith-Wiedemann	Macroglossia, organomegaly, macrosomia, ear creases, omphalocele
Fragile X	Macrosomia, mental retardation, language disorder, macroorchidism, abnormal connective tissue
Hemihypertrophy	Similar to Beckwith-Wiedemann, but only one side of the body is macrosomic
Marshall-Smith	Macrosomia, characteristic faces with shallow orbits, wide middle finger, accelerated skeletal growth
Sotos	Macrosomia, delayed development, large hands and feet, dyscoordination
Weaver	Macrosomia, characteristic faces, accelerated skeletal growth, camptodactyly

half of the body is macrosomic. Babies with hemihypertrophy have the same complications of prolonged hypoglycemia and increased tumorgenesis that occurs in Beckwith-Wiedemann. If children with these two syndromes survive infancy, ultrasonic examinations of the abdomen should be ordered every 3 to 6 months to check for neuroblastomas and Wilm's tumors.

Rarer still than Beckwith-Wiedemann and hemihypertrophy are the other syndromes listed in Table 22.3. These various syndromes are not related to each other except for the common factor of increased pancreatic secretion of growth-inducing hormones and neonatal prolonged hypoglycemia. Table 22.4 provides information about infants at risk for hypoglycemia.

The causes of s*mall for gestational age* (SGA) babies (less than 2200 g or 4 lb, 13 oz at term) are more varied than for LGA babies. The causes for SGA babies are summarized in Table 22.5.

Do not forget that a major cause of SGA babies is normal-sized premature babies with an incorrect expected date of confinement (EDC). Much less common than in the preultrasound era, a baby can still be 4 or even 8 weeks less mature than predicted because of dating mistakes.

In general, small parents have small babies; however, the reasons parents are small are both varied and complex. Adults may be small because of genetic factors, poor protein nutrition before their birth, poor protein nutrition after their birth, or a combination of these reasons. A multigenerational study of Japanese immigrants to Hawaii was

Table 22.4 Infants at risk for hypoglycemia

Maternal history of diabetes
Maternal medications:
- Tocolytic agents
- Steroids
- Oral antidiabetic agents
- Illicit drugs

Neonatal factors:
- Prematurity—gestational age <37 wk
- 5-min Apgar ≤5 (infants who have been resuscitated)
- SGA or <2500-g weight
- LGA or >4000-g weight
- Discordant twins >400-g difference

Maternal history of untreated endocrine deficiencies or excesses
Maternal history of untreated metabolic disorders
Neonates known to have abnormal chromosomes
- Example: trisomy 21; XXY; XO

Clinical findings of hypoglycemia:
- Tremors, jitteriness, irritability
- Hypertonia, hypotonia
- High-pitched, weak cry
- Eye rolling, staring, or other signs of seizure activity
- Lethargy and/or poor feeding
- Cyanosis/apneic spells
- Pallor, hypothermia
- Cardiomegaly, cardiac failure
- Difficulties with waking

Note: Hypoglycemia in the newborn can be present with or without symptoms. The presence of symptoms does not always indicate the severity of the hypoglycemia.

conducted between the 1860s and 1960s. This Japanese population was insular and did not marry outside the community until the fifth generation. The original immigrants had an average adult height for men of under 5 ft 2 in. and for women of under 4 ft 10 in., due to chronic protein malnutrition. It was not until the fourth generation that the average adult heights in this population had risen to reach the same size as the rest of the Hawaiian population. From this study, one can see that an acquired trait (short stature because of chronic protein malnourishment) was in some sense passed on in an increasingly weakening effect to four generations. This same gradual move toward the United States norm for height has been seen in other protein-starved immigrant populations

Table 22.5   Primary causes of small for gestational age (SGA) infants

- Decreased nutrition/oxygen flow through placenta
- Small maternal size (primarily height)
- Infection
- Congenital growth retardation syndromes (rare)

such as Ashkenazi Jews and will probably be seen in the current group of Southeast Asians.

Any process that diminishes blood flow or oxygenation of the placenta, and thus of the baby, will diminish birth size. Poor maternal diet, especially if there is a significant lack of calories or protein, will decrease infant size. Table 22.6 lists causes of poor nutrition in utera. Processes occurring throughout the pregnancy, such as maternal smoking, cause symmetrical retardation of length, weight, and head circumference, while processes occurring late in pregnancy (preeclampsia, for example), mainly affect weight. Some of the causes of SGA show unusual patterns of poor growth—alcohol, especially, causes severe microcephaly. The most common causes of growth retardation in utero from infection are the TORCH infections (see Chapter 11).

Table 22.6   Causes of poor nutrition in utero

Hypoxia

- Living at high altitude
- Maternal smoking
- Maternal profound anemia
- Maternal chronic pulmonary disease
- Congenital hypoxic heart disease

Poor maternal nutrition
- Mothers <15 years old
- Mothers >40 years old
- Mothers not eating enough calories or enough protein
- Maternal smoking
- Abuse of alcohol
- Abuse of illicit drugs associated with anorexia

Poor vascular flow to the infant
- Long-standing maternal diabetes
- Chronic maternal hypertension
- Poor placental implantation
- Collagen vascular diseases such as lupus

Table 22.7   Congenital syndromes of microsomia

Disease	Symptoms/Signs
All abnormalities of chromosome number except multiple Xs	
Cornelia de Lange	Catlike cry in infancy, slow bone growth, severe mental retardation, synophrys (fused eyebrows) with very bushy eyebrows
Russell-Silver	Very small, normal head circumference, asymmetric bones, normal intelligence
Seckel	Very short, microcephalic, large nose, frequent MR, 11 pairs of ribs
Williams	Small, prominent lips, MR, hoarse voice, vavular heart disease, disorders of calcium
Osteochondrodysplasias	All are collagen defects, Achondroplasia is the most common and least lethal with the classic short limbs, especially proximally, low nasal bridge, apparent macrocephaly

In standard texts of congenital defects, there are several hundred named dwarfing syndromes. In Table 22.7, the most common are listed. Achondoplasia and trisomy 21 (Down syndrome) are much more common than the others in this list (each presenting in slightly less than 1 in 200 babies).

Chapter 7 discusses hypoglycemia in the delivery room. A more detailed list of babies at risk for hypoglycemia can be found in Table 22.4. Chapter 7 also discusses the controversy over how to define hypoglycemia, concluding it is as 45 mg/dL or less. After the first 8 hours of life, the practitioner should attempt to keep all newborns' serum glucose levels above 60 mg/dL.

SUGGESTED READING

Jones, KL. *Smith's recognizable patterns of human malformation,* 5th ed. Philadelphia: WB Saunders, 1997.

CHAPTER 23

Newborn Hearing Screening

Gary A. Emmett

The current cost of funding a child with true hearing loss is greater than $25,000.

Figure 23.1 provides a pathway for newborn hearing screening. Newborn hearing screening is recommended by the American Academy of Pediatrics (AAP) and is mandatory now in many states. Discovering congenital hearing loss and treating it before 6 months of age markedly improves long-term outcomes. The problem with screening is that the rate of congenital hearing loss in the United States is very low, making its cost effectiveness seem low.

In 2000, 73% of the hospitals and birthing centers in the United States and its territories reported at least a limited program of hearing screening. Approximately 65% of newborns were reportedly screened, although the actual number screened may have been higher. Follow-up was erratic, with less than 100% follow-up in most localities. The Centers for Disease Control and Prevention (CDC) recorded that 56% of the 21,000 babies referred for follow-up hearing screen evaluations in the year 2000 were actually tested. The CDC states that the actual follow-up percentile may be higher, because reporting mechanisms varied from state to state and also in quality of reports. In data reported to the CDC, less than 10% of the referred babies had significant hearing loss and were enrolled in an early intervention program. As chapter is being written, there are no long-term follow-ups to see what the results of these interventions were. The actual rate of hearing loss in newborns is very close to the previously estimated rate, which was about 1 in 1,000.

When a program first starts, 5% of the newborns tested will have an abnormal screen, with only 1 out of 50 actually having hearing loss. As programs mature, the specificity of the test increases with increased operator experience, and this rate goes from 5% to under 2%. In both new and mature programs, the number of children with actual hearing loss stays at about 0.1%. This low incidence of true-positives presents many problems for the well nursery practitioner. The major dilemma is how not to frighten the parents whose infants have positive tests, because most of them will have normal hearing, but to strongly encourage them to return for a follow-up examination in 2 weeks.

After the second test, there will still be more false-positives than true-positives found, but children who have failed the test twice should be referred to the ear, nose, and throat (ENT) and/or speech department for an Auditory Evoked Response test. Of true-positive hearing loss, 70% of cases have a genetic basis, and 30% are of an unknown or infectious origin.

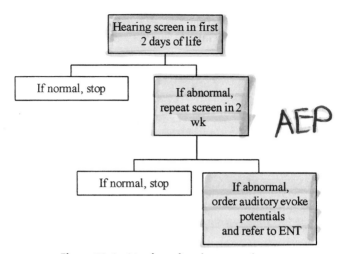

Figure 23.1   Newborn hearing screening.

Convincing all initially abnormal screens to return for follow-up testing is challenging. The hospital and/or the practitioner must have a consistent system so that deaf children are not lost to follow-up. Once a child is known to be deaf, the challenge is to determine which pathway in deaf education the child should take. Educators of the deaf are deeply divided over whether sign language or "total language" should prevail; what is clear, however, is that any treatment is better than no treatment.

Hearing loss can occur at any time during life. Just because a child passes its birth hearing test, do not assume the child can hear well. If a child has marked delay in speech acquisition, or does not respond to loud noises, please continue to do hearing testing when appropriate.

SUGGESTED READING

Centers for Disease Control and Prevention. Infants tested for hearing loss—United States, 1999–2001. *MMWR,* 2003 Oct 17;52:981–984.

Circumcision

Judith Turow, Jay Goldberg and Erika Johnston

*Circumcision is highly controversial.
Many strong opinions in both directions
seem to be based more on emotions than
on fact. The editor believes that the
complications of the procedure and the
disease states avoided by the procedure
are economically and physically about
equal. Therefore, circumcision is purely a
social decision. We have two views of
circumcision, the first by a pediatrician,
and the second, with a practical review
of how to do a circumcision, by
two obstetricians.*

JUDITH TUROW, MD

In circumcision, the foreskin is surgically separated from the penile glans and then partially or wholly removed. In utero, the penile skin grows forward to completely cover the glans. Initially, there is no separation between the squamous epithelium covering the glans and the foreskin. If left alone, separation of the glans and the foreskin usually occurs between 2 and 5 years, and the foreskin will retract naturally by the end of puberty.

Circumcision is a personal decision that is made for a variety of social, religious, and medical reasons. The practitioner should ask the parents about their feelings on circumcision. See Fig. 24.1. If the parents do not want a circumcision, it should not be done. The only diseases that necessitate a circumcision are phimosis, paraphimosis, and balanitis, which are rare to nonexistent in newborns. Phimosis, or the inability to retract the foreskin, should never be diagnosed before the third birthday, because the foreskin is not retractable until that time. Paraphimosis, the trapping of the foreskin below the glans, is usually caused by trying to retract a nonretractile foreskin. This condition may lead to a surgical emergency, because ischemia of the glans can occur with subsequent

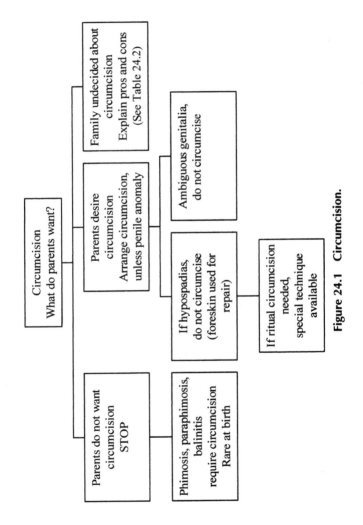

Figure 24.1 Circumcision.

Table 24.1   Conditions canceling/postponing circumcision

Canceling
- Abnormal appearing genitalia (except for undescended testicles)
- Inability to determine phenotype of child (ambiguous genitalia)
- Less than 12 hours of age (physiologic adaptation requires 12 to 24 hr)
- Severe illness or suspected infection
- Constitutional small penis (micropenis, <2.5 cm from pubic bone to tip of glands)

Postponing
- Active sepsis workup
- Delayed voiding (no urination since birth)
- Family history of bleeding disorder
- Ingestion of formula within 30 min of circumcision
- Small penis due to prematurity
- Significant illness

tissue destruction. The foreskin should not be retracted before the third birthday because of the possibility of paraphimosis. Balanitis is an infection of the foreskin, and if recurrent, some recommend circumcision.

If the parents desire a circumcision, the practitioner should make arrangements. Either the pediatric practitioner or the obstetrician will do routine circumcisions, as per local custom. Some parents request a ritual circumcision, and this procedure may be arranged by the parents themselves.

Table 24.1 lists conditions canceling or postponing circumcision. Some newborn males should never have a circumcision. If a child has ambiguous genitalia, a circumcision should be postponed until the child's true sex and sex of rearing are determined. If the child has a hypospadias (ventral misplacement of the urethral opening), epispadias (dorsal misplacement of the urethral opening), and/or chordee (congenital fixed curvature of the penis), then circumcision should be postponed, because the foreskin is used in repair of these anomalies. In these cases, a ritual circumcision can be performed that draws only one drop of blood and does not remove any tissue. The circumcisions of sick and premature babies should be postponed until they are completely stable. In most hospitals, circumcisions are postponed if the child is undergoing a sepsis workup or treatment, even if the child is not ill at the usual time of circumcision. If the child has a family history of a bleeding disorder, the circumcision should be postponed until the diagnostic labs are done.

If parents are undecided about a circumcision, the practitioner must explain the reasons for and against the procedure without letting his or

Table 24.2   Circumcision discussion points

Arguments against circumcision include:
- Cost—$300 per baby (average in 2002). The total cost of circumcision in the United States in 2002 was close to half a billion dollars.
- Complications—rare and usually minor (see Table 24.3).
- Pain—newborns do experience pain. Analgesia is strongly recommended before circumcision (discussed in Dr. Goldberg's article).
- Decrease in penile sensation—articles argue both for and against this idea. The true answer is not known.
- Decreased immune function—this argument is not sustained in the literature.
- Ethics—is it right to perform a permanent change in the baby's bodily functions without the baby's consent?

Arguments for circumcision include:
- Social norms—baby should look like his father.
- Religious norms—male circumcision is required by both Judaism and Islam; other social/religious groups may encourage circumcision.
- Urinary sepsis in the first month of life—circumcision lowers rate of urinary tract infection in first year of life from 14 per 1,000 to 2 per 1,000.
- Decreased chance of acquiring sexually transmitted diseases (STDs) including HIV—true, but not significant compared to lifestyle issues.
- Penile cancer prevention—only true if patient is circumcised as child.
- Penile hygiene—probably no more effective than cleanliness.

her personal feeling influence the discussion. Table 24.2 lists discussion points.

If a circumcision is done, pain relief may be proved by surgical analgesia, as discussed later. In addition, methods of pain relief include acetominophen (15 mg per kg per dose every 6 hours), sweet wine by mouth, and breast-feeding after the procedure. All have been shown to markedly reduce the child's pain. Documentation of both the child's degree of pain and the practitioner's alleviation of that pain should be recorded in the child's medical record.

The child usually stays in the hospital for at least several hours after circumcision to allow for the clot to solidify. Some hospitals require the infant to urinate before discharge, but this precaution is not medically necessary. Usually a gauze wrap is placed around the penis. This can be removed 24 hours after the circumcision. If the gauze is difficult to remove, it should be wet with water. When a child is circumcised, it is common for the parent to see a white-yellow secretion around the site for about 5 to 7 days. Direct the parent to keep the circumcision scar clean with plain water, never alcohol, and cover the area with a lubricant such as Vaseline or A&D Ointment. Sometimes a plastic ring is used instead of gauze; this ring takes 5 to 8 days to drop off.

Two natural processes often mistaken by the parents for complications of circumcision are adhesions and smegma. In circumcised males, adhesions are linear white elevated scarlike lesions arising at the base of the glans that are formed by the epithelium. Parents should be reassured that these are normal. In uncircumcised males, smegma are the skin cells shed as the foreskin and glans separate in the second to fifth year of life. Smegma is white and shiny and is often mistaken for infection of the foreskin. Smegma can be gently cleaned off with water and a washcloth. Infection of the foreskin involves erythema, warmth, and swelling, which are not present if the discharge is simply smegma.

JAY GOLDBERG AND ERIKA JOHNSTON

Newborn male circumcision is defined as the intentional surgical removal of the male penile foreskin. The incidence of infant male circumcision has significantly decreased over the last 20 years. Although an estimated 80% of infant males were circumcised in 1980, reportedly only 64% had the procedure performed in 1995. Circumcision is still the third most commonly performed surgical procedure in this country, with over one million annually.

Absolute contradictions to circumcision are listed in Table 24.1. A relative contraindication to circumcision is a child greater than 6 to 8 weeks of age. By this age, more adhesions may have formed, causing the procedure to be more difficult and time consuming, possibly requiring a more experienced clinician. The foreskin may also develop significant edema after lysis of these adhesions. By this age, maternally contributed clotting factors may also have been used up, which, possibly, increases the risk of bleeding.

Complications of circumcision are listed in Table 24.3. Gynecologists believe that after bleeding, meatal stenosis is the most common complication of circumcision. It results from contraction of the meatus following healing of the inflamed, denuded glans or from damage to the frenular artery at the time of circumcision. A narrowing pronounced enough to cause deflection of the urinary stream, or dysuria, requires a corrective meatotomy. Removal of insufficient foreskin or inner preputial skin may necessitate redoing the circumcision.

Circumcision of male infants normally should be discussed with the parents before birth at obstetrical visits or birthing classes. If a decision has not been made, a postpartum discussion is also necessary. Written consent should be obtained and placed in the infant's chart,

Table 24.3   Complications of circumcision

Complication	Incident	Treatment
Bleeding	>1%	Pressure, rarely cautery
Infection	>0.4%	Appropriate antibiotics (cephalexin 50 mg/kg daily, divided QID)
Dehiscence	>0.16%	Local care
Denudation of the shaft	>0.05%	Local care
Glandular injury	>0.02%	Local care

Other, more rare, complications:
- Concealed penis
- Unsatisfactory appearance
- Interference with urination
- Meatal stenosis
- Complete amputation of the penis
- Incomplete circumcision

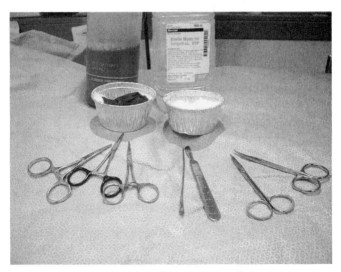

Figure 24.2   Materials and sterile instruments necessary for circumcision. From left to right in foreground: hemostats × 3, probe, scalpel, straight scissors, curved scissors; in background: betadine solution, sterile water, and cotton swabs in aluminum dishes.

as for any surgical procedure. Risks of the procedure listed should include infection, bleeding, and damage to the penis requiring additional surgery.

Jewish parents may elect to have a religious circumcision for their male infants, a *bris* or *Brit Milah*. The *bris* is normally performed on the eighth day of life, with the day of birth counting as the first day if the child was born before sundown. The *mohel*, or religious practitioner of circumcision, should be knowledgeable regarding both surgical technique and Jewish law, as documented by a certifying board.

Figure 24.2 shows the materials and instruments needed for circumcision. Without analgesia, circumcised newborns experience more pain and stress as measured by changes in heart rate, blood pressure, oxygen saturation, and cortisol levels. The American Academy of Pediatrics states that analgesia is safe and effective in reducing the pain associated with circumcision and should be used if the procedure is performed. Surgical analgesia includes the following:

- topical analgesic creams,

- dorsal penile nerve block, and

- subcutaneous ring block.

The most commonly used topical analgesia for circumcision is eutectic mixture of lidocaine/prilocaine analgesia (EMLA) cream, a mixture

Table 24.4   Penile dorsal nerve block

Equipment needed:
- 1% lidocaine without epinephrine
- 1 cc syringe with 27-gauge needle
- Alcohol pads

Technique:
- Using sterile technique, draw up 1 cc of 1% lidocaine without epinephrine in a 1 cc 27-gauge tuberculin syringe.
- Cleanse the penis and skin surrounding the genitals.
- Stabilize the penis with gentle traction. If the umbilicus marks the 12 o'clock position, insert the needle at the 2 o'clock position to a depth of 0.5 cm beneath the skin surface. Taking care not to inject intravascularly (check by aspirating), inject 0.5 cc of 1% lidocaine without epinepherine. Repeat the injection at the 10 o'clock position. Do not exceed a total of 1 cc of lidocaine.
- Anesthesia will be optimal after 2 to 3 minutes. Thus, for time efficiency, perform the penile block prior to setting up the circumcision set.

Table 24.5   Gomco circumcision

1. After identifying the infant, restrain him using the infant board.
2. Inspect the penis for abnormalities.
3. Anesthetize the penis.
4. Using alcohol or other antiseptic solution, clean an area about 3 in. in diameter around the base of the penis and the entire penis.
5. (When describing the penis, the dorsum will be described as the 12 o'clock position.) Using hemostats, grasp the edge of the foreskin at points between the 2 o'clock and 3 o'clock positions and again between the 9 o'clock and 10 o'clock positions. Take care not to clamp the hemostats onto the glans. Place gentle upward traction on the foreskin. Gently insert a straight hemostat or probe between the foreskin and the glans to the depth of the corona, at the 12 o'clock position. Sweep in both directions toward the ventral attachment of the foreskin to the glans, separating adhesions between the glans and foreskin. Be careful not to extend beyond the depth of the corona or traumatize the urethra.
6. While lifting the foreskin away from the glans, firmly clamp the dorsal aspect of the foreskin, using a straight hemostat to a depth of about one third of the total distance to the corona.
7. Remove the straight hemostat.
8. While tenting the skin, carefully cut along the center of the clamp line, being careful not to extend beyond the line of crushed tissue.
9. Gently retract the foreskin from the glans.
10. Inspect the glans and foreskin for remaining adhesions. Gently separate any residual adhesions, using either a probe, hemostat, or gauze.
11. Place the bell of the Gomco clamp over the glans. We prefer using the 1.1 Gomco for most circumcisions, unless the penis is larger than normal.
12. Manipulate the foreskin using the curved hemostats (still attached) while applying gentle downward pressure on the handle of the Gomco bell, to pull the foreskin over the bell. The protective bell should be between the glans and the foreskin, set against the corona.
13. Grasp and reapproximate the two sides of the foreskin with a hemostat around the shaft just above the Gomco bell.
14. With gentle traction in a distal direction, insert the distal end of the Gomco bell, hemostat, and foreskin completely through the opening in the body of the Gomco clamp. Clamp the bell on to the Gomco and tighten slightly.
15. Check for appropriate placement of the Gomco and the foreskin. The foreskin should be drawn through the body of the Gomco circumferentially even. The apex of the initial incision should be

(continued)

Table 24.5   (*Continued*)

visible, above the Gomco body. When the Gomco clamp has been appropriately positioned, firmly tighten it.

16. With a scalpel cutting against the bell of the Gomco, incise the foreskin to remove the distal portion.
17. Unclamp the Gomco, removing the body and clamp of the Gomco.
18. To separate the bell from the penis, gently press with a moistened piece of cotton gauze.
19. To control any bleeding, first apply pressure. For persistent bleeding, silver nitrate or Gelfoam can be applied to hasten clotting. If continued bleeding requires suturing, use a small absorbable suture. Persistent bleeding after circumcision is a common sign of factor-deficient bleeding disorders, such as hemophilia. If bleeding is refractory to these measures, clotting studies and a hematology consultation should be considered.
20. Wipe off excess antiseptic with a moist gauze to prevent a local skin reaction. Place white petrolatum and gauze (or a piece of white petrolatum gauze) over the penis and rediaper.
21. Document the time of day in the chart. The infant should not be discharged until he has voided.

of local anesthetics 2.5% lidocaine and 2.5% prilocaine. This formulation has been found safe from concerns about local irritation, uneven absorption, or systemic toxicity. ELMA has been shown in a double-blind, randomized, controlled trial, to decrease crying and heart rate increases compared to placebo during circumcision. EMLA, to work effectively, needs to be applied to the penis 1 hour prior to the circumcision. Given the often-unpredictable schedule of an obstetrician or pediatrician, this time frame may be the biggest obstacle in routinely using topical analgesia for circumcision. Details of penile dorsal nerve block are found in Table 24.4. Details of the subcutaneous ring block can be found in any standard obstetrical text.

The most common circumcision techniques are the Gomco, Mogen, and PlastiBell. All techniques give equivalent results. The choice of which to use is largely based on the operator's method of training and personal preference. We describe all three techniques. For Gomco, see Table 24.5 and Fig. 24.3 and 24.4; for Mogen, see Table 24.6 and Fig. 24.5; and for PlastiBell, see Table 24.7.

If postcircumcision bleeding occurs, it is normally controllable through holding direct pressure on the penis for several minutes. If this is unsuccessful, other options include cauterizing the bleeding area by applying silver nitrate or Monsel's solution. Occasionally, the area must be sutured. This should be performed superficially using a 4.0-caliber absorbable suture. The occurrence of resistant bleeding should raise the suspicion for and initiate the evaluation of a possible bleeding disorder.

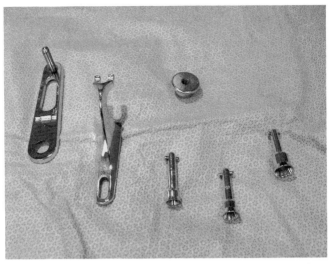

Figure 24.3 Gomco disassembled with bell sizes (left to right).

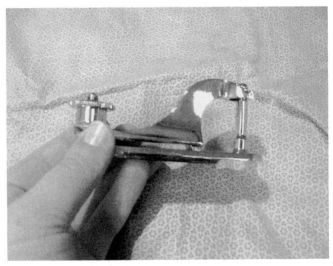

Figure 24.4 Gomco assembled.

Table 24.6   Mogen method

Technique

1. As in steps 1 through 9 of the Gomco method, identify and restrain the infant, inspect the penis for abnormalities, cleanse the area, and separate the glans and foreskin.
2. Further separate any remaining adhesions.
3. Use the hemostats to pull the foreskin tight. Horizontally, place the Mogen clamp over the foreskin. Advance the clamp proximally until the appropriate amount of foreskin is distal to the clamp. After verifying that the tip of the glans is not within the clamp, tighten the clamp.
4. Use the scalpel to excise the foreskin flush against the distal edge of the Mogen clamp.
5. Remove the clamp.
6. Gently separate the foreskin, exposing the glans of the penis.
7. As in steps 19 through 21 of the Gomco method, check for bleeding, cover with petrolatum gauze, and rediaper.

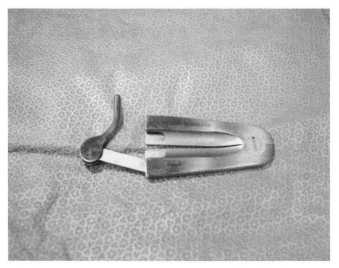

Figure 24.5   Mogen clamp assembled.

Table 24.7   PlastiBell method

Technique
1. As in steps 1 through 3 of the Gomco method, restrain the infant, inspect the penis for abnormalities, and administer anesthesia.
2. As in steps 4 through 10 of the Gomco method, cleanse the area, separate the foreskin from the glans, tent the tissue, clamp and remove the hemostat, cut along the hemostat line, retract the foreskin, and break down any remaining adhesions. While the hemostat is clamped, loosely place the PlastiBell string (2-inch diameter) around the base of the penis and put two turns in the string.
3. Place the PlastiBell over the glans and pull the foreskin over it.
4. Remove one hemostat and hold both sides of the foreskin with a single hemostat.
5. Position the PlastiBell so that the indentation is below the apex of the incision and at the appropriate place on the foreskin. Use the hemostat to clamp across the shaft of the PlastiBell and hold the other hemostat to keep the foreskin in this relationship.
6. Place the string over the PlastiBell's indentation, tightening the string until it just remains in place.
7. Check placement of the string and bell again, ensuring that the apex of the foreskin incision is distal to the string, so that excessive skin is not being removed.
8. Tighten the string as much as possible, holding tension for 30 seconds. Tie a square knot in the string.
9. Remove the hemostats.
10. Cut the foreskin to within 1/8 to 3/16 in. distal to the string.
11. Trim the ends of the string to 1/2-in. long.
12. While stabilizing the body of the PlastiBell, gently bend the shaft of the PlastiBell with the other hand until it snaps at the junction of the bell and the shaft.
13. The PlastiBell should be able to move up and down on the glans.

As in steps 19 through 21 of the Gomco method, check for bleeding, cover with petrolatum gauze, and rediaper.

SUGGESTED READING

Lerman SE, Liao JC. Neonatal circumcision. *Pediatr Clin North Am* 2001;48:1539–1557.

American Academy of Pediatrics. Circumcision policy statement. *Pediatrics* 1999;103:686–693.

Pfenninger JL. *Procedures for primary care physicians.* St. Louis, MO: Mosby, 1995.

CHAPTER 25

Delayed Stooling

William B. Stephenson

If a newborn has not stooled in the first 24 hours of life, successfully taking a rectal temperature will rule out anal atresia and avoid embarrassment for everyone.

Delayed passage of the first meconium stool is an important indicator of newborn gastrointestinal dysfunction. Figure 25.1 provides pathways for delayed stooling. Delayed passage of stool, which is defined as first stooling after 24 hours of age, can result from congenital disease, anatomic lesions, motility disorders, endocrine disorders, and electrolyte disturbances. Approximately 27% of infants will stool in the delivery room, and by 24 hours of age, 92% of infants will have passed meconium.

Normal stooling is widely variant. Some infants have only one stool per day, especially those on formula feeding. Others may stool with each feeding. Such frequent stooling is common in breast-fed infants during the first month of life. Initially, stools are extremely viscous and dark green in color. This meconium stool is usually gone by 48 hours of age. After 24 hours, a mixture of meconium and regular stool, called a transitional stool, is evident. Bottle-fed babies have a dark brown to light green stool that is formed but soft. Breast-fed babies have a light brown to bright yellow stool that is primarily liquid in consistency, with light brown "seeds" in each stool. Infants should not have hard, rocklike stools or stools that contain either fresh (red) or old (black) blood. Microscopic blood in the stool is normal in babies, both because of swallowed maternal blood at the time of delivery and, if breast-feeding, because of cracking and bleeding of mothers' nipples. Straining with stools is normal in newborns and does not imply pathology. Table 25.1 provides some stooling definitions.

To determine if infants with delayed stooling have pathology, a thorough history and careful physical examination are essential. Most important is confirming that the report of delayed stooling is true. A close review of all delivery records and nursery records, and discussion with all the infant's caregivers, may reveal that the child has indeed passed meconium, but the passage has not been documented.

A physical examination that reveals a generally ill newborn without specific findings should lead to an immediate rule-out sepsis workup. Necrotizing enterocolitis presents a similar picture, except that the child usually has a tender and distended abdomen. Simple examination often finds anal disorders such as atresia, stenosis, or anterior displacement. If any anal disorders are identified, a further imaging evaluation

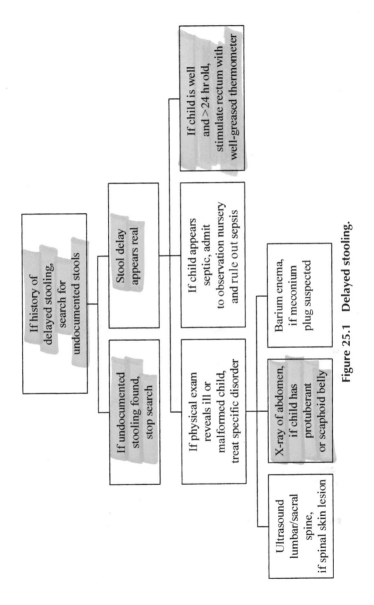

Figure 25.1 Delayed stooling.

Table 25.1   Some stooling definitions

Delayed stooling	*Arbitrarily* defined as no stools by 24 hr of age
Meconium	Thick, dark green, viscous matter that has accumulated in the child's gut while in utero, primarily made from the defoliated skin cells and skin secretions of the fetus
Meconium plug	Compressed meconium that is very dry and causes a distal impaction of the bowel

for elements of the CHARGE and VATER syndromes (cardiovascular malformations, skeletal malformations—especially hemivertebrae and abnormal radii, renal and urogenital dysplasia, and esophageal disruption) should be undertaken. The spine should be examined for skin defects that may indicate spina bifida occulta, because malfunction in the sacral nerves may prevent the relaxation of the internal sphincter in response to a full rectal vault. Ultrasound of the spine is a very safe method in the nursery if an external abnormality of the spinal cord is noted. Table 25.2 lists causes of delayed stooling.

A flat plate of the abdomen is useful if the child appears obstructed. Stenosis, atresia, or duplication of the gut will cause obstruction, as

Table 25.2   Causes of delayed stooling

- Physiologic delayed stooling
- Necrotizing enterocolitis
- Malformations of the anus
    (Look for other malformations of CHARGE or VATER syndromes
        Cardiovascular malformations
        Esophagial disruption
        Skeletal malformations
        Urologic dysplasia)
- Spinal malformations
- Obstruction/duplication of bowel
- Meconium plug
        Cystic fibrosis
        Hirschsprung's disease
- Metabolic disorders
        Congenital hypothyroidism
        DiGeorge syndrome
        Hypermagnesemia
        Hypocalcemia
        Infant of diabetic mother
        Maternal hyperparathyroidism

will toxic megacolon, necrotizing enterocolitis, or neonatal small left colon syndrome. Toxic megacolon is a massive dilatation of the distal colon associated with Hirschsprung's disease (an aganglionic segment of the distal colon). Necrotizing enterocolitis is most frequently seen in anoxic, ill newborns, but this necrosis of the gut wall can occur in any infant. Infants of diabetic mothers may be found to have a neonatal small left colon, which resolves spontaneously.

A barium enema can be both therapeutic and diagnostic. A meconium plug may be evacuated by the barium. Approximately 20% to 30% of infants with a meconium plug will have Hirschsprung's disease. However, in the newborn period a barium enema may not be diagnostic for Hirschsprung's, because the transition zone between ganglionic and aganglionic segments is not sharp. If bowel dysmotility continues, a suction biopsy for ganglion cells in the colon is warranted. Ten to 15% of children with cystic fibrosis will present with a neonatal meconium plug. Any child with a meconium plug and no obvious cause should be given a sweat test.

Metabolic disorders may also result in delayed stooling. Hypocalcemia may delay stool and is seen in infants of diabetic mothers, maternal hyperparathyroidism, and DiGeorge syndrome (22q11 deletion). If the DiGeorge syndrome is suspected, a chest X-ray is warranted to assess for rib abnormalities and absence of a thymus. Hypermagnesemia typically results from magnesium given to the infant's mother to control high blood pressure, but may result in a very constipated baby. Congenital hypothyroidism can also result in chronic constipation.

If no obvious pathology can be found, simple stimulation of the rectum with a well-lubricated rectal thermometer may induce the first stool. Occasionally no obvious cause of delayed stooling can be found, but the child will start stooling late and continue stooling uneventfully. In these cases, no further workup is warranted.

SUGGESTED READING

Fanaroff AA, Martin RJ (Ed). *Neonatal-perinatal medicine: diseases of the fetus and infant,* 7th ed., Vol. 2. St. Louis, MO: Mosby, 2002, 1269–1289.

Sherry S, Kramer I. The time of passage of the first stool and first urine by the newborn infant. *J Pediatr* 1955;46:158–159.

Delayed Urine Output

William B. Stephenson

Not urinating in the first 24 hours is less likely than not recording that urination.

Adequate urine output in the infant indicates adequate intravascular volume, good oral intake, and a normally functioning genitourinary system. In healthy term infants, approximately 17% will urinate in the delivery room and 92% will urinate in the first 24 hours. The definition of adequate urine output in a newborn is the first urination by 24 hours of life and then at least three diaper-soaking urinations per 24 hours thereafter. Figure 26.1 provides pathways for delayed urination in the newborn.

If a newborn is not urinating, all caregivers need to be interviewed about possible undocumented urination. Caregivers should also be asked about the child's oral intake, although the exact definition of adequate oral intake in the first 24 hours of life is not clear. If poor documentation does not appear to be the cause of the child's anuria, consider the prenatal course of the infant. Did the child have oligohydramniosis? In severe oligohydramniosis, the lack of amniotic fluid may deform the child severely, resulting eventually in Potter's facies (widely separated eyes, low-set ears, and receding chin). If severe enough, oligohydramnios will lead to hypoplastic lungs and probable death. Causes of oligohydramniosis include bilateral renal agenesis and posterior urethral valves. Placental insufficiency caused by placental abruption, preeclampsia, other causes of poor blood flow to the infant, or fetal maternal transfusion may lead to a fluid-depleted infant at birth. A review of prenatal records, especially renal ultrasounds, is warranted. Lack of amniotic fluid may also be associated with rupture of membranes, maternal group B *Streptococcus* colonization, or other genital infections. Table 26.1 lists causes of anuria in the newborn.

As in any ill child, a physical examination may be revealing. The child should be examined for dry mouth, absence of tears, and poor vascular return. If the practitioner believes the child is mildly dehydrated, then extra formula may be dripped into the baby's mouth. If the baby is unstable to take oral fluids, an IV should be started, a fluid bolus should be given, and the child should be transferred to a monitored bed.

In stable infants, the oropharynx should be examined for hard and soft palate defects and for a weak suck. Infants should be observed while feeding to determine if the suck is coordinated and efficient. In some breast-fed infants whose mothers have short nipples, an inferior lingual frenulum can interfere with proper feeding and must be clipped. All these abnormalities can complicate feeding and can lead to inadequate oral intake.

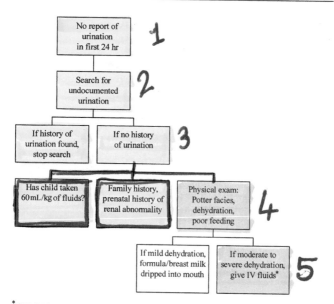

*If IV fluids are needed, give a bolus of 10 to 20 mL/kg of normal saline over ½ hr and then about 120 mL/kg per 24 hr of ¼ normal saline with potassium added once the child urinates

Figure 26.1 Delayed urination in newborn algorithm.

The abdominal exam can reveal sinus tracts, fistulas, and abdominal masses. It may also reveal an obstruction that prevents proper hydration.

Genital malformations are common sources of urinary malfunction. In males, urethral stricture, hypospadius, epispadius, and phimosis should be readily evident and may be associated with a weak urinary stream. In females, the exam is more difficult. The possibility of bladder fistulas to the vagina and rectum are possible, and diapers should be checked for abnormally wet stool and caregivers asked about vaginal discharge.

Table 26.1	Causes of anuria in the newborn

Anuria or oliguria in the newborn results from:

- Poor infant oral intake (minimum 60 mL/kg first 24 hr, 80 mL/kg second 24 hr, 100 mL/kg per 24 hr thereafter)
- Congenital kidney dysfunction
- Obstruction of urine outflow

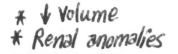

Imaging studies are useful and required in children with possible urinary tract disease. An ultrasound of the urinary tract should be done in any child with a history of delayed first urination. A voiding cysturethrogram (VCUG) may reveal several conditions and is diagnostic if one suspects bilateral urethral valves. Ultrasound of the spine is performed in those cases where a sacral spinal abnormality leads to suspicion of a tethered cord interfering with normal bladder function.

If the child is otherwise stable, simple observation may be employed for the first 36 hours of life. If the infant is mildly dehydrated or having difficulty latching on, the infant can be fed either pumped breast milk or formula by dropper to restore/maintain hydration. If no urine output has occurred by 36 hours, the bladder should be catheterized to prove urine is being produced. At that time, serum electrolytes, blood urea nitrogen, and creatinine should also be obtained to demonstrate the functional status of the kidneys. Remember: The newborn's electrolytes up to 48 hours of age may reflect the mother's electrolytes.

SUGGESTED READING

Sherry N, Kramer I. The time of passage of the first stool and first urine by the newborn infant. *J Pediatr* 1955;46:158–159.

Avery G, Fletcher M, MacDonald M. *Neonatology: pathophysiology and management of the newborn,* 5th ed. Philadelphia: Lippincott Williams and Wilkins, 1999:755–757.

* RUS

* VCUG

CHAPTER 27

Discharge

Judith Turow

Careful wording of the last words the practitioner says before discharge can save a life.

Appropriate discharge of the newborn from the hospital requires education of the caregiver and assessment of the newborn by the pediatric practitioner. See Fig. 27.1. The caregiver must know how to recognize the child's needs and appropriately respond to them. He or she must also be taught to recognize when the child is seriously ill. Assessment of the baby by the pediatric practitioner includes recognizing any significant disease and probable complications after the child leaves the hospital. Problems such as gastrointestinal obstructions, ductus dependent cardiac lesions, and jaundice often take several days to develop. The practitioner must assess the health of the child, the health of the mother, and the social relationship between them. Newborns should not

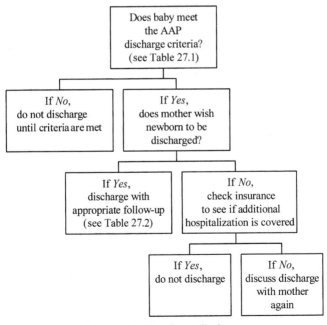

Figure 27.1   Newborn discharge.

Table 27.1   AAP/ACOG minimal criteria for a short-stay (<2 day) discharge of a healthy newborn

The following minimal criteria should be met before a newborn is discharged from the hospital after an uncomplicated pregnancy, labor, and delivery.

1. The antepartum, intrapartum, and postpartum for both mother and neonate are uncomplicated.
2. Delivery was vaginal.
3. Single AGA birth at 38–42 wk of gestation (see Fig. 21.5)
4. At discharge, the baby has just had 12 hr of stable vital signs, including a respiratory rate below 60/min, a heart rate of 100 to 160 beats per min, and the ability to maintain a body temperature in an open crib with typical newborn clothing of 36.1–37.0°C.
5. The baby has urinated and passed at least one stool.
6. The baby has finished at least two successful feedings, and it is documented that it can suck, swallow, and breathe while feeding. If breast-feeding, an actual feeding should be observed by a knowledgeable caregiver.
7. Physical examination shows no abnormalities that require continued hospitalization.
8. If circumcised, there was no evidence of excessive bleeding at the site for at least 2 hr.
9. There is no visible jaundice in the first 24 hr of life *(the editor strongly believes that all children should have a percutaneous or serum bilirubin measurement prior to discharge).*
10. The mother's (or preferably both parents') knowledge, ability, and confidence to provide adequate care for the neonate are documented by the fact that the following training and information have been received.
    - Condition of the neonate
    - The breast-feeding mother–neonate dyad should be assisted by trained staff regarding nursing position, latch on, and adequacy of swallowing
    - Knowledge of appropriate urine and stool frequency
    - Umbilical cord, skin, and infant genital care
    - Temperature assessment and use of thermometer
    - Recognition of illness, particularly jaundice
    - Instruction in proper newborn safety, including use of a car seat and BACK TO SLEEP
11. Support people such as family members or health care providers are available to the mother to discuss newborn's care, lactation, jaundice, and dehydration in the first few days after discharge.
12. Parents know what instructions to follow in the event of a complication or emergency.

(continued)

Table 27.1   (*Continued*)

13. Laboratory data are available and reviewed, including maternal syphilis, hepatitis B virus surface antigen, HIV status, cord or infant blood type, and direct Coombs' test if indicated.
14. Screening tests are performed in accordance with state regulations. If the test is performed before 24 hr of milk feeding, a system for repeating the test is to be ensured during the follow-up visit.
15. Initial hepatitis B vaccine is administered or a scheduled appointment for its administration has been made within the first week of life.
16. A source of continuing medical care for the mother and baby is identified.
17. A definite appointment is made for the baby to be examined within 48 hr. The follow-up visit can be made in the home or office, as long as the person evaluating the newborn is knowledgeable and competent about newborns, and reports the results of the visit to the family doctor or designee.
18. Family, environmental, and social risk factors have been discussed as well as assets. When risk factors are present, the discharge should be delayed until they are resolved or a plan to safeguard the newborn is in place. Factors include but are not limited to
    • Untreated parental substance abuse or positive urine toxicology test in mother
    • Past history of child abuse or neglect
    • Mental illness in a parent
    • Lack of social support
    • Lack of fixed home
    • History of untreated domestic violence
    • Adolescent mother

be discharged from the hospital until the child is medically stable and the parents are aware of their child's needs.

In October 1995, the American Academy of Pediatrics (AAP) came out with a statement of what they believed were the minimum requirements for a term newborn to be discharged at less than 48 hours. This statement was revised in 2002. The AAP recommended that the mother and child be discharged simultaneously, if possible. Although early discharge was a trend driven by parents in the 1980s, financial considerations pushed an even wider application of this trend in the 1990s. There is no convincing data that hospitalization of 48 hours or more is better than a hospitalization of 24 hours or less. Achievement of successful parent/child outcomes such as breast-feeding, positive mother–child interaction, and firm bonding clearly take different amounts of time in different mothers and children. Mother–neonate dyads may successfully

Table 27.2   Model newborn discharge instructions

The next few weeks will be a growing experience for you and your baby as you get to know each other. Relax, trust your instincts, and enjoy the moments. The following instructions review the most frequently asked questions.

Call your baby's doctor if:

1. *Fever,* in the first six weeks of life, of greater than 100.0°F (take temperature under the baby's arm)
2. Baby does not make *urine at least three* times and have at least *one bowel movement* every 24 hours. They can have many more. Follow the breast-feeding log book to make sure your baby is urinating and stooling enough every day.
3. Your bottle-feeding baby has *waterlike* or *bloody bowel movements.*
4. Your breast-feeding baby has *bloody bowel movements.* In breast-fed babies, very loose stools with yellow seeds are normal.
5. *Diaper rash* that does not seem to be getting better in 2 to 3 days
6. Persistent *vomiting.*
7. *Irritable, sluggish,* or *unable to arouse* for feedings during the day.
8. *Shortness of breath* or *color changes* on the face while feeding.
9. *Feeding much less* than what is usual for your baby.
10. *Redness of skin, persistent drainage, or worsening of foul smell* around the base of the umbilical cord.
11. *Increasing yellow tone* to skin or whites of eyes.

Trust your judgment—you know your baby better than anyone else.

WHEN IN DOUBT, CHECK IT OUT!

Important telephone numbers
1. Baby's doctor _____
2. Police 911 or your local medical emergency phone number _____

Feeding
1. Allow your baby to eat when he or she becomes hungry.
2. Some feeding cues that your baby is hungry are *fussiness, wakefulness, putting hands to face, or sucking on hands.*
3. Babies may want to feed as often as every 2 hours. Babies sometimes cluster their feedings together. *Breast-fed babies* may eat as often as every hour.
4. If your baby is sleeping 3 to 4 hours during the daytime, you may want to wake him or her for a feeding.

Bath—Sponge bathe the baby until the umbilical cord falls off (usually by 14 to 21 days of age). When the cord has been completely off for 24 hours, you may then tub bathe your baby.

(continued)

Table 27.2   (*Continued*)

Umbilical cord—Keep the cord *dry* and cleanse the base of the cord with alcohol 3–4 times per day until it falls off. You may apply alcohol to the belly button for 1–2 days after it falls off to ensure complete drying of the area.

Circumcision—Apply A&D Ointment to the tip of the penis for 3–4 days at each diaper change until it is healed.

Safety/Security
1. Everyone should *wash* his or her hands before holding or caring for your baby.
2. Place your baby on his or her *back* or side to sleep.
3. Always place your baby in a *car seat,* which is buckled in the back seat facing the rear of the vehicle. Follow the car seat manufacturer's instructions for correct installation of the car seat.
4. *Never* shake your baby!
5. To be comfortable, babies always need one more thin layer of clothing than their parents.
6. To protect your infant from possible home abduction (kidnapping), the following guidelines are recommended:
   a. Never let anyone you don't know into your home without identification. This includes home care nurses and doctors.
   b. Outdoor decorations on your home advertising the birth of your baby are not recommended; however, if they are used, they should be taken down later that same day.
   c. Birth announcements in the newspaper/television/internet should not include your home address.

Your baby's blood tests
At the time of discharge, your baby was checked for many birth problems that could harm him or her if not treated. These test results will come back within the next 2 weeks. It is *vital* that you provide your nurse with an accurate home address and a phone number where you can be contacted in the event that your infant's tests are abnormal. The lab will contact you, the hospital, and your baby's doctor. Make sure that they can *contact you*. If any of the newborn blood tests were taken when the baby had not been feeding for at least 24 hours, the test should be repeated on your first visit to the doctor or nurse.

Hearing Screen
Your baby's hearing was screened while he or she was in the hospital. About 1 in 50 babies fail this screening test, but very few of these children have a hearing loss. The problem is, we don't know which children who fail these tests have hearing problems and which ones do not. It is *essential*, if your baby has failed this test, that you follow up in 2 to 3 weeks with a hearing center to make sure that everything is normal.

Follow-up appointment: _____

Medications: _____

be discharged before 24 hours if properly prepared. Table 27.1 gives the minimum criteria felt necessary by the AAP (in association with the American College of Obstetrics and Gynecology, ACOG) for a short hospitalization (less than 48 hours) in a healthy term newborn. At many institutions, a serum or percutaneous bilirubin level is also required prior to discharge. Appropriate follow-up of hyperbilirubinemia is found in Chapter 33.

When the practitioner and the mother both feel that the mother and child(ren) are ready for discharge, clear instructions must be given to the parents. Among the instructions, parents must be told that if a child is less than 48 hours of age, early follow-up by either a home visit or an office visit for the baby within 2 to 3 days is strongly recommended. In addition, if the child has been fed for less than 24 hours, the hospital/practitioner must make arrangements to repeat the newborn metabolic screen as an outpatient.

The practitioner is concerned about many problems that may occur after discharge. A model hospital discharge list given to the mother and explained to her by the nursing staff is found in Table 27.2. Because of their frequency in causing immediate problems, three specific areas should be emphasized. The child must urinate at least three times every 24 hours and have at least one bowel movement. This demonstrates that the child is being adequately fed. If the child feels warm, the caregiver must take the child's temperature. If the rectal temperature is greater than 100.4°F or 38°C, this is a medical emergency, and the primary practitioner must be immediately informed. The parents should look at the whites of the child's eyes and skin daily in the sunlight, and if they observe increased jaundice, they should call the primary practitioner and have it checked as soon as possible.

SUGGESTED READING

American Academy of Pediatrics/American College of Obstetrics and Gynecology (AAP/ACOG). *Guidelines for perinatal care,* 5th ed. Elk Grove Village, IL: AAP; Washington, DC: ACOG, 2002.

CHAPTER 28
Newborn Metabolic Screening
Gary A. Emmett

Newborn metabolic screens help prevent permanent damage to children from many inborn errors of metabolism, but they also open up a Pandora's box of difficult ethics and privacy questions; specifically, how much we should know about each individual's genetic makeup and who is allowed access to that knowledge.

Starting with the newborn test for phenylketonuria (PKU) 40 years ago, we have gradually increased the number of tests in the newborn screen. There is no national minimum number of screening tests, but all states check for PKU, hypothyroidism, hemoglobinopathy, and classical galactosemia. Two-thirds of the states in the United States check for congenital adrenal hyperplasia and maple syrup urine disease. Some states test for as many as 37 metabolic illnesses. At this moment, the technology for diseases that result in a single small molecule in abnormal amounts is quite inexpensive. So with ten or twelve drops of the baby's blood, the first test may cost $5 or $10 or $15, but each subsequent test added on will cost only a few pennies. Some congenital metabolic diseases that respond well to a screening program are not screened, such as alpha$_1$-antitrypsin deficiency, because they produce only an abnormal protein, and large molecules are at present expensive to screen. With new advances in technology, the cost of inquiring about these enzymatic diseases may be markedly less expensive in the near future.

In most states, the statewide screening program takes responsibility for finding newborns with abnormal screening tests. These agencies usually have the ability to both track down the patient and refer them to community-wide special programs in their defect. But, the practitioner who receives notice of an incomplete or abnormal test is still responsible for attempting to contact the parents and should note the follow-up into the patient's chart or into a special newborn metabolic screening file. Table 28.1 was obtained from the newborn screening test center of the State of Pennsylvania, which has a large optional screening program in addition to the basic six tests.

Table 28.1 Disorders detectable by supplemental newborn screening

Disorder	Treatment	Outcome Treated	Outcome Untreated
Argininosuccinic-aciduria	Protein-restricted diet.	Frequent metabolic crises precipitated by excessive protein intake, fever, or infections.	Death.
Citrullinemia	Protein-restricted diet.	Frequent metabolic crises precipitated by excessive protein intake, fever, or infections.	Death.
Homocystinuria	Methionine restriction for early detection and pyridoxine treatment for later detection.	Prevention or long-term delay of symptoms.	Mental retardation, eye dislocation, high mortality from blood clots. Approximately 50% die by age of 25.
Hypermethioninemia	Methionine restriction for early detection and pyridoxine treatment for later detection.	*Elevated blood levels of methionine is not a disease but a marker of other diseases especially homocystinuria and tyrosinemia.*	
Maple syrup urine disease	Dietary restriction of branched chain amino acids requiring a special formula; intensive monitoring of status, especially during stress and illness.	Children who are monitored closely and supported during metabolic crises are doing well.	Death.

Phenylketonuria	Lifelong dietary management.	Functionally normal to near normal.	Mental retardation, eye dislocation, high mortality from blood clots. Approximately 50% die by age of 25.
Tyrosinemia type I	Dietary restriction of tyrosine and phenylalanine with special formulas.	Stabilizes the liver disease and ameliorates the kidney, bone, and CNS symptoms, but organ failure may still occur in severe cases. Liver cancer remains a risk. Liver transplants will cure.	Death from liver failure or hepatocellular carcinoma.
Tyrosinemia type II	Dietary restriction of tyrosine and phenylalanine with special formulas.	Skin and eye manifestations resolve, and neurological impairment is minimized.	Skin and eye manifestations, along with mental retardation.
Tyrosinemia type III	Breast milk or commercial formula similar to breast milk and ascorbic acid should be given. Treatment should continue for several weeks.	No long-term sequellae.	Initial symptoms can be quite serious.
3-hydroxy 3-methylglutaryl-CoA lyase deficiency	Leucine-restricted diet and supplemental glucose to prevent hypoglycemia. Dietary supplementation with carnitine may be warranted.	Patients appear to be well and to develop satisfactorily.	Death during childhood.

(continued)

Table 28.1 (*Continued*)

Disorder	Treatment	Outcome Treated	Outcome Untreated
Glutaricacidemia type I	Intravenous fluids and bicarbonate are used to treat acidosis; dialysis may be necessary. Protein-restricted diet. Riboflavin and carnitine supplementation.	Neurologic status is stabilized, and future complications are usually prevented. Early treatment may allow for normal development.	Results in varying degrees of neurologic impairment from mild to marked dystonia and rigidity. A few patients remain asymptomatic.
Isovalericacidemia	Correct dehydration, electrolyte disturbances, and metabolic acidosis. Exchange transfusion, hemodialysis, and peritoneal dialysis may be needed. Give adequate caloric intake with IV glucose to reverse catabolic state. Reduce protein intake, remove excess isovaleric acid by administering glycine and carnitine, reduce blood ammonia.	Overall prognosis depends on the severity of the enzyme deficiency and management of the initial and subsequent acute episodes. If well managed, patients can have a relatively normal life. Treatments are vastly improving overall outcomes.	Death soon after birth.
2-methylbutyryl-CoA dehydrogenase deficiency	Protein restriction with restricted isoleucine intake.	Unknown. May depend on genetic and environmental background.	

(continued)

	Treatment	Outcome
3-methylcrotonyl CoA hydratase deficiency	Dietary restrictions. Supplementation with carnitine and/or biotin.	
3-methylglutaconyl-CoA hydratase deficiency	Low-protein diet and limiting leucine content may be useful. Carnitine supplementation has helped some patients.	
Methylmalonic-acidemia	Protein restricted diet. Cobalamin and L-carnitine supplementation. If carnitine is not helpful, restrict isoleucine, theonine, methionine, and valine. Dialysis may be required for severe ketoacidosis and hyperammonemia.	Brain damage, including coma, generalized seizures, and death.
Propionicacidemia	Acute episodes are treated by correcting dehydration, electrolyte disturbances, and metabolic acidosis. Peritoneal dialysis to remove ketoacids and ammonia. Chronic management includes a protein-restricted diet and prophylactic antibiotics, as well as supplementation with L-carnitine and biotin.	Normal development is possible, but most patients have some degree of permanent neurodevelopmental deficit despite adequate therapy.
Carnitine/acylcarnitine translocase deficiency	Treat hyperammonemia and cardiac problems first. Avoid fasting. Supplement with oral carnitine, low fat diet, frequent feedings.	Originally thought to be uniformly fatal, but recent studies show that patients with milder variants survive and stabilize after the neonatal period. Early death.

Table 28.1 (*Continued*)

Disorder	Treatment	Outcome Treated	Outcome Untreated
Carnitine palmityl-transferase II deficiency	Treat hyperammonemia and cardiac problems first. Avoid fasting. Supplement with oral carnitine, low-fat diet, frequent feedings. Late-onset form is treated by avoiding both fasting and prolonged exercise.	Late-onset form is generally not fatal.	Neonatal presenting forms are often fatal.
3-hydroxy long-chain acyl-CoA dehydrogenase deficiency and trifunctional protein deficiency	Low-fat, high-carbohydrate diet, medium-chain triglyceride supplementation. Frequent meals. Support with glucose during intercurrent illnesses.	More than two-thirds of patients are alive and doing well with treatment.	Without treatment, 75%–90% of patients die.
Medium-chain acyl-CoA dehydrogenase deficiency	Low-fat diet with adequate calories. Frequent feeding. Avoid fasting and support aggressively with glucose during infectious episodes. Carnitine supplementation.	Aggressive support during illness has greatly reduced morbidity and mortality. As children get older, they have fewer crises.	Without treatment, 25% of children died, and 37% of those surviving had significant developmental problems.

Multiple acyl-CoA dehydrogenase deficiency or glutaricacidemia type II	Frequent meals with night feeding, if a severe form. Low-fat and low-protein diet. Riboflavin supplementation aids some patients, especially late-onset types.	Late-onset patients do well if supported during stress and if fed frequently to avoid crises.	Usually fatal during early life.
Short-chain acyl-CoA dehydrogenase deficiency	No standard treatment is available.		Too few cases to make conclusions.
Short-chain-hydroxyacyl CoA dehydrogenase deficiency	None established. Too few cases.		Unknown. Generally fatal if symptomatic as infants.
Very long chain acyl-CoA dehydrogenase deficiency	Low-fat diet with frequent feedings. Avoid fasting. Medium-chain triglyceride supplementation to replace long-chain fatty acids.	Few metabolic crises, stabilized or even improved myopathy and cardiopathy. Well-managed patients do well.	Recurrent and potentially fatal acute metabolic crises, heart failure from cardiomyopathy. Carnitine supplementa-
Mitochondrial acetoacetyl CoA thiolase deficiency	Sodium bicarbonate and intravenous fluids for acidosis. Dialysis may be needed. Carnitine supplementation has been helpful in some cases.		

(continued)

151

Table 28.1 *(Continued)*

Disorder	Treatment	Outcome Treated	Outcome Untreated
Arginase deficiency	An essential amino acid– and arginine-free diet. Benzoate and phenylacetate may also be helpful.	Too few patients to determine outcome.	Progressive spastic quadriplegia, seizures, developmental delay, mental retardation, irritability, hyperactivity.
Biotinidase deficiency	5 to 10 mg of oral biotin per day.	All symptomatic children improve. In some treated children, all symptoms resolve, whereas in others deficits are irreversible.	Neurological and cutaneous findings that include seizures, hypotonia, and rash, often accompanied by hyperventilation, laryngeal stridor, and apnea.
Multiple CoA carboxylase deficiency	Oral biotin supplementation to begin immediately on diagnosis.		

Congenital adrenal hyperplasis due to 21-α-hydroxylase deficiency	Cortisol replacement. In the severe form, the salt-retaining hormone aldosterone must be replaced by the drug Florinef. Antiandrogen agents are being evaluated to control excessive virilization. Females should be surgically corrected to be as anatomically appropriate as possible.	Treated patients generally have normal lives except that they may be short in stature. Even females with masculinization that has been corrected have borne children.	The severe male patients can die before they are diagnosed. Females are usually noticed because they are born with ambiguous genitalia and are treated.
Cystic fibrosis	Most patients attend a CF center where they are evaluated quarterly by a multidisciplinary team consisting of physicians, nurses, respiratory therapists, dietitians, social workers, and genetic counselors.	Increased life spans and better quality of life.	Death in teenage years.
Galactosemia	Lactose-galactose–restricted diet	If diet is provided during the first 10 days of life, the presenting symptoms quickly resolve and the complications of liver, sepsis, neonatal death, and mental retardation can be prevented. However, children with galactosemia remain at risk for developmental delays, speech problems, and abnormalities of motor function.	Feeding problems, failure to thrive, hepatocellular damage, and sepsis.

(continued)

Table 28.1 (Continued)

Disorder	Treatment	Outcome Treated	Outcome Untreated
Galactokinase deficiency	Dietary treatment is the same as that for classical galactosemia.	Intellectually normal. No cataracts.	Cataracts.
Galactose-4-epimerase deficiency	Asymptomatic form treatment is low-galactose diet. Children with the generalized epimerase deficiency are placed on a galatose-free diet.	Generalized epimerase deficiency—mental retardation. Asymptomatic patients are always normal.	Generalized epimerase deficiency—cataracts, jaundice, and hyperbilirubinemia.
Glucose-6-phosphate dehydrogenase deficiency	Avoid certain medications including antimalarials, methylene blue, sulfonamides, phenacetin. Avoid substances including fava beans, naphthalene, quinine. Use common cold, allergy, or cough medications with caution.	No problems.	Fair; growth problems, learning difficulties, anemia, and jaundice.

Carbamoyl-phosphate synthetase deficiency	Protein-restricted diet and medications to increase nitrogen excretion. Dialysis may also be required.	There is a good prognosis if the disorder is treated prospectively from birth.	Newborn presentation generally is catastrophic in nature and leads to rapid demise without rapid recognition and treatment. 100% mortality if untreated. There is a direct correlation between the duration of hyperammonemic coma and mental retardation, developmental delays, and cortical atrophy.
Carnitine palmitoyl-transferase I deficiency	Frequent feeding of low-fat diet and use of medium chain triglycerides. Glucose infusions should be used to support during minor illnesses that could precipitate crises.	Excellent with treatment.	Patients can have neurological deficits.
2,4-dienoyl-CoA reductase deficiency	None to date.	—	Only patient identified was a neonatal death.

(continued)

Table 28.1 (*Continued*)

Disorder	Treatment	Outcome Treated	Outcome Untreated
5-oxoprolinuria (pyroglutamic-aciduria)	Avoidance of drugs and oxidants that may cause hemolysis. Avoidance of stressors such as infection and surgery. Metabolic acidosis is treated with IV bicarbonate. Supplement with antioxidants such as cysteine, penicillamine, mercapto-pyridoxal, and vitamin E.	Unknown	—
Hyperornithinemia-hyperammonemia-homocitrullinuria syndrome	Protein restriction. In patients with ornithine transporter defect, ornithine, arginine, or citrulline supplementation have been effective.	Because underlying cause is known, hyperammonemia can be better managed. As a result, patients are expected to be less effected.	Delayed development, choreoathetosis, seizures, and low intelligence.
Gyrate atrophy	No standardized therapy, but the goal is lower plasma ornithine levels.	Not well managed by known treatments.	Most patients have a progressive disorder leading to total blindness.

Malonic aciduria	A low-fat, high-carbohydrate diet. Hospital admission is recommended during periods of infection, as well as during febrile illness to manage hypoglycemia.	No hypoglycemic episodes.	Developmental delay, seizures, hypotonia, diarrhea, vomiting, metabolic acidosis, hypoglycemia, ketosis, and lacticacidemia.
Ornithine transcarba-moylase deficiency	Protein-restricted diet and medications to increase nitrogen excretion. Dialysis may also be required.	There is a good prognosis if the disorder is treated prospectively from birth.	100% mortality if untreated. There is direct correlation between the duration of hyperammonemic coma and mental retardation, developmental delays, and cortical atrophy.

SUGGESTED READING

Genetic and newborn screening resource center of the US (NNSRC). http://genes-r-us.uthscsa.edu (2003 Nov 21).

Part IV

After Discharge

CHAPTER 29

Practitioner Responsibilities After Hospital Discharge

Gary A. Emmett

Discharge planning starts at the moment of hospital admission.

Unfortunately for the well nursery practitioner, his or her responsibilities do not stop with the signing of the discharge order. The hospital practitioner is responsible for the welfare of the newborn until a relationship is established between the newborn's caregivers and his or her primary care practitioner. Therefore, during each newborn hospital stay, three areas of postdischarge care must be discussed:

1. Does the newborn have a primary care practitioner?

2. Do the parents have a safe physical environment for the child after discharge?

3. Are there appropriate caregivers for the child after discharge?

Figure 29.1 provides pathways for the practitioner's responsibilities after the child's discharge from the hospital.

As stated in chapter 27, a newborn is expected to have posthospital follow-up within 72 hours. Although second and subsequent children in the family, especially if they are bottle-feeding, are often not seen for up to 2 weeks, all discharge planning should assume that follow-up will be as soon as possible. On the first hospital visit to the mother, the practitioner should ask the name of the primary care follow-up. If the mother does not have a practitioner for the child, then there should be a list available of qualified pediatricians and family practitioners in areas served by the hospital's maternity service so that the mother may choose the most appropriate one.

Sometimes, the parents are unable to find a primary care practitioner who will accept their infant because of financial or insurance reasons. The hospital practitioner must maintain a service for these infants for the first month of life. It does not matter whether the practitioner personally maintains an outpatient service or just maintains a close relationship with an outpatient service, as long as a service is available to provide follow-up for all newborns for the first month of life. In most jurisdictions, the baby is covered by the mother's insurance for that period.

Other times, the family is unable to find a practitioner because of a long, complicated neonatal hospital course. Many primary caregivers are appropriately uncomfortable with the close follow-up of these patients. In addition to the well baby posthospital practice described

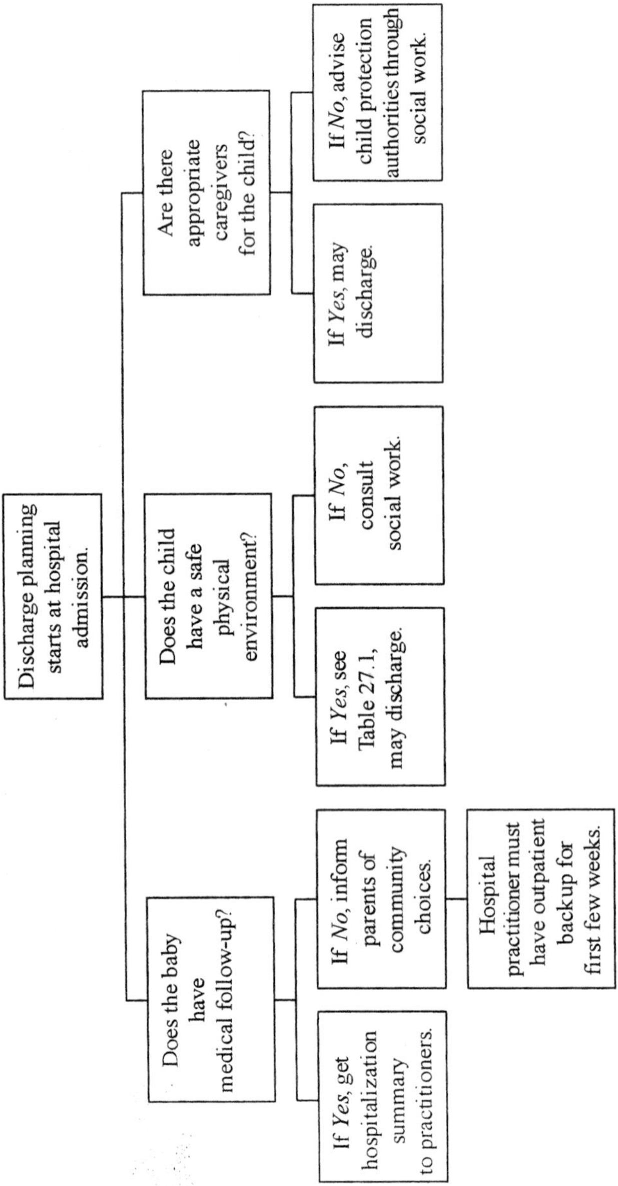

Figure 29.1   Practitioner's responsibilities after newborn hospital discharge.

earlier, the hospital practitioner must have a high-risk follow-up program available for the ill or very premature child discharged from the nursery. Chapter 38 discusses the high-risk follow-up clinic in greater detail.

After establishing medical care for the newborn follow-up, the hospital practitioner should inquire about some minimal environmental standards that should be met before a child is discharged. Primarily, there must be a safe home for the child. Sometimes there is not even a home for the child to go to. If homelessness can be identified early in the newborn hospital course, then the social work team has time to find an appropriate posthospital environment for the newborn. For physical standards, see Table 29.1.

The car seat is a vital part of the home environment checklist. No baby should go home except in an adequate car seat. Many hospitals will not discharge a baby without a car seat being present. For the first year of life, the car seat should be placed facing backward in the second or third row of seats. The seat must also be properly secured according to the manufacturer's installation instructions. Improper installation is the number one reason for problems with infant car seats.

In children born at less than 37 weeks, authorities believe that apnea can occur in many car seats. Some hospitals, following the 1990 American Academy of Pediatrics policy, require a car seat test using the car seat in which the baby will go home. See Table 29.2 for criteria for properly performing a car seat test for the premature. In 2003, a New Zealand group found that the simple insertion of a soft headrest would allow most prematures to travel safely in a car seat.

Table 29.1   Newborn home environment checklist

Safe home available	
Adequate car seat	If <37 weeks, do premature car seat testing
Available nutrition	If unable to attain food, WIC may be available
Safe crib or bassinet	Bassinet adequate until child weighs at least 12 lb or can turn over
No pillows	
Firm bedding	
Only firm toys	>2 inches across at narrowest diameter
Bars closer together than width of head	<$3^{1}/_{2}$ in. on center
Adequate clothes for climate	One thin layer more than necessary for adults
Smoke alarms in child's bedroom	

Table 29.2   Testing car seat for premature newborn

- Position patient in the car seat that the premature infant will use.
- Infant should be reclining with harness fastened and retainer clip on chest.
- Attach child to pulse, respiration, and oxygen saturation monitor system.
- Record for full 90 min.
- Significant events:

Desaturation	<90%
Apnea	>20 sec
Bradycardia	<80 beats/min

- If significant events persist, stop test.
- If significant events occur during test, or if test has to be stopped, the test is considered a failure.
- If failure:

  Test can be repeated every 24 hours *or*

  Child can go home in a child safety bed (available from Cosco, Inc.)

Finally, the pediatric practitioner who sees the mother and child in the hospital should attempt to establish whether there is an adequate caregiver environment for the newborn after discharge. Sometimes the parents are unable to care for the child because of personal problems such as mental illness, substance abuse, a previous history of child neglect or abuse, or a current incarceration. Any alternate family caregiver should be approved by the hospital social work department that can help place the child in a safe environment.

All three of these discharge criteria should be documented on the newborn chart, in addition to being discussed with the parents. An absolute necessity that must be clearly documented on the chart at the time of discharge is a current working phone number and a mailing address. Even if the parents do not have a phone or clear mailing address, they must have a friend, relative, or neighbor with a phone and the ability to contact them quickly. Emergencies will arise that need follow-up, such as an inadvertent infectious disease exposure, an inadequate or abnormal newborn screening result, and bilirubin follow-up.

The home visits provided by many insurance plans and public health departments can be an important asset following newborn discharge. In most cases, the visits can assess the well-being of the mother and the child and the adequacy of the home environment. Although in some cases no diagnostic criteria are needed for home visits, in almost all situations the infant can be followed up for inadequate growth and hyperbilirubinemia. The standard criterion for adequate newborn nutrition is a weight loss of 9% or less while in the hospital. The criteria for bilirubin follow-up are listed in Table 15.4.

SUGGESTED READING

American Academy of Pediatrics/American College of Obstetrics and Gynecology (AAP/ACOG). *Guidelines for perinatal care,* 5th ed. Elk Grove Village, IL: AAP; Washington, DC: ACOG, 2002.

AAP Committee on Injury and Poison Prevention and Committee on Fetus and Newborn. Safe transportation of premature infants. *Pediatrics* 1991;87:120–122.

Tonkin SL, McIntosh CG, Hadden W, Dakin C, Rowley S, Gunn AJ. Simple car seat insert to prevent upper airway narrowing in premature infants: a pilot study. *Pediatrics* 2003;112:907–913.

Significant Events during Car Seat test :-

① Apnea ⩾ 20 Seconds

② HR < 80/min

③ Desat. < 90%

C H A P T E R   30
First Outpatient Visit
Gary A. Emmett

*The first office visit completes the
process of transition. The practitioner
tries to resolve all of the well
nursery issues.*

During the first office visit, the practitioner attempts to resolve all of
the issues in the transition from in utero life to postnatal existence. In
addition to the routine physical and the question of whether the family is
adjusting well to the new addition, a short series of important questions
must be answered. These are listed in Table 30.1.

Is the baby gaining weight? Almost all newborns lose weight after
birth; the fetus is almost 90% water, whereas the child is only 80% water.
This water loss accounts for much of the change in weight immediately
after birth. During the first 2 days after birth, an infant will lose 3% to
9% of its birth weight. In a large baby of 4,500 gm (9 lb 15 oz), this
loss can amount to almost a pound.

In judging weight in the newborn, knowing both the birth weight
and the discharge weight is essential. A breast-fed infant loses more
weight and takes longer to get back to birth weight, but any full-term
infant should be back to birth weight by the tenth day of age. Babies are
expected to gain a minimum of 15 g per day and may gain as much as
60 g a day. The average newborn weight gain is 25 g per day. Because
25 g is almost 1 oz, over a short period of time, a baby can be expected
to gain 1 oz per day.

After weighing the naked baby, one subtracts the discharge weight
from the current weight and divides the difference by the number of
days since discharge. If this number shows a gain of at least 15 g ($^1/_2$ oz)
per day, then no further weights need be done until the next scheduled
visit. If the child has not gained 15 g per day but is not losing weight,
then the baby should be weighed again in 1 week. If the baby has lost
weight since discharge, then detailed questions must be asked about the
feeding process, the number of urinations per day, and the number of
bowel movements per day. Table 30.2 lists causes of weight loss by the
first visit.

Can the parents calm the baby? In the normal course of a new infant's
life, the cycle of eating, stooling, sleeping, and then waking up crying
for more food occurs every 2 to 6 hours. If the child cannot be calmed by
the parents, and also cannot be calmed in your office, that may warn of
serious underlying disease. Metabolic disease, ischemic heart disease,
and even cow's milk protein allergy may make the child extremely
irritable. A more complete list of causes of irritability may be found in
Table 30.3. Calming techniques may be found in Table 30.4.

Table 30.1	Important questions at first visit

- Is the baby gaining weight?
- Can the parents calm the baby?
- Is the infant alert?

Table 30.2	Causes of failure to thrive

- Inadequate feeding:
    Bottle: <2 oz/lb or 4 oz/kg per 24 hr
    Breast: no feeling of fullness or dripping in mother
    Child not urinating TID
    Child not having at least one daily bowel movement
- Congenital heart disease
    Is the baby short of breath with feedings?
    Is the back edematous?
- Metabolic defect
    Is newborn screen normal?
    Does child have reducing substances in urine?
    Does baby have a peculiar odor?
- Inadequate emotional support
    Is the baby being held?
    Are the parents interacting with the baby?
- Hyperthyroidism
    Bradycardia?
    Cool skin?
    Poor interpersonal interaction?

[handwritten annotation: 4 oz/Kg/day]

Table 30.3	Causes of prolonged irritability

All causes of failure to thrive except hyperthyroidism (Table 30.2)
- Trauma, including bleeding in brain (from birth or from shaken baby syndrome) or bone fracture
- Ligature around body part, especially fingers, toes, or penis (frequently caused by long, fine hair)
- Hepatitis
- Pancreatitis
- Obstruction of urinary system
- Anomolous origin of coronary vessels (they arise from the pulmonic artery instead of the aorta)

Table 30.4   Calming techniques

Feeding	No sooner then every 2 hr breast-feeding or 3 hr bottle-feeding.
Nonnutritional sucking	Pacifiers are not accepted by every baby, but do not cause damage to teeth until the baby has teeth. Breasts are also used as pacifiers if acceptable to mother.
Papoosing	Newborns do not, in general, like being in open spaces. By firmly wrapping a blanket around a child, many children can be calmed.
Rhythmic sounds	Loud clocks, metronomes, and music with a consistent beat will calm many children.
Motion	Carriage rides, car rides, being carried over a walking parent's left shoulder, or just leaning against a washing machine with a child is very soothing to the newborn. Inexpensive devices are available that rhythmically shake the crib and make a repetitive sound at the same time, combining these last two actions.

Last, is the infant alert? If the child does not focus on its parent's eyes and follow them regularly, one must seriously consider encephalopathy and/or seizures.

CHAPTER 31

Immunizations

Gary A. Emmett

Immunizations are one of the fundamentals of pediatric practice. We should inform the parents about the importance and frequency of immunizations before they leave the well baby nursery.

The only immunization regularly given in the well nursery is the first hepatitis B vaccine. As you can see from Chapter 13, it is vitally important that if the mother has hepatitis B, her child be vaccinated as soon after birth as possible. But why do we give it to everyone? First, laboratories can make mistakes, and you do not want to miss any parent with hepatitis B who might then give it to their newborn child: 25% of babies who acquire hepatitis B soon after birth will eventually develop liver cancer. Second, it is extremely important to prevent hepatitis B for everyone. Most people acquire hepatitis B after they become sexually active, but it is very difficult to give immunizations to adolescents and young adults.

In Britain in the 1980s, the National Health Service attempted to give the rubella vaccine only to postpubertal females to minimize potential side effects. This process seemed to make sense, because rubella or German measles is an extremely mild illness in children and is dangerous only when a mother contracts it during pregnancy. In many places in the world, rubella is still the most common cause of congenital deafness. Unfortunately, even with a system where immunization and health care are free, Britain could never get more than 25% of adolescent females immunized and therefore could not stop rubella from attacking fetuses and making them deaf.

The program in the United States, where rubella was given at 15 months and at 4 years, was markedly more effective. By eliminating German measles in school children, the United States eliminated German measles in pregnant women, because there was no longer a reservoir of disease available. Giving the rubella vaccine to males, who will not directly benefit from it, may lead to ethical quandaries, but it works for the general population. In the same manner, babies are relatively easy to immunize, and we have effectively eliminated the acquisition of hepatitis B among a whole generation of Americans by giving them their immunization a decade or two before they would ever need to use it.

Figure 31.1 is the 2003 Centers for Disease Control and Prevention (CDC) approved immunization guideline. Because this information

169

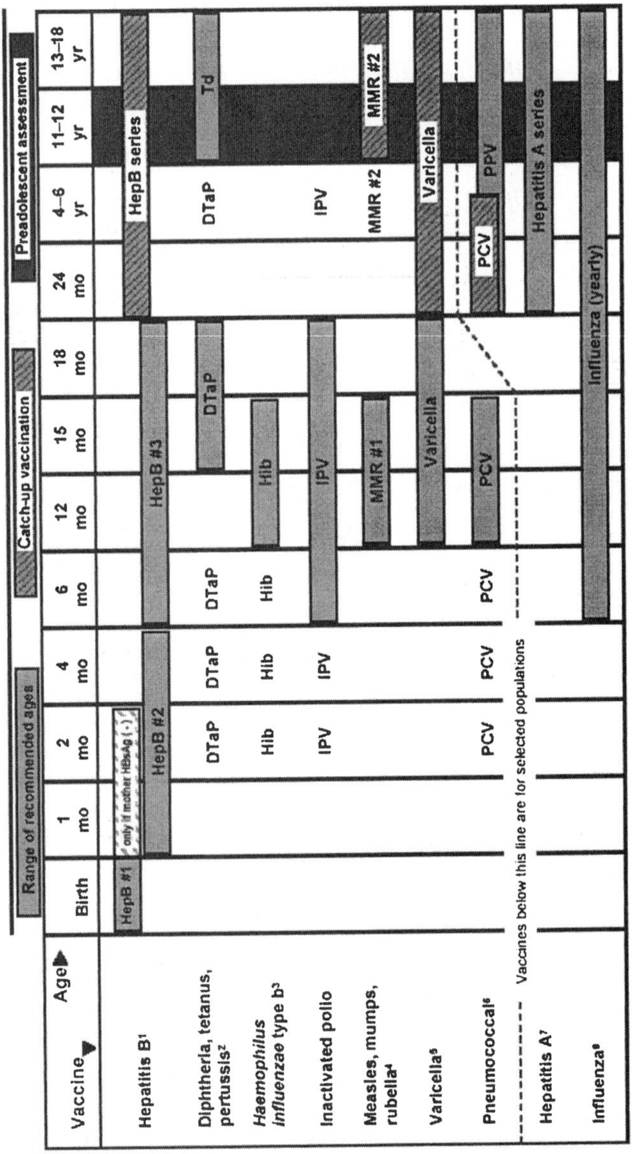

Figure 31.1 CDC childhood immunization schedule.

changes rapidly, please consult the CDC immunization webpage, which is currently at http://www.cdc.gov/nip/recs/child-schedule.PDF, to get the latest information.

This schedule indicates the recommended ages for routine administration of currently licensed childhood vaccines, as of December 1, 2002, for children through age 18 years. Any dose not given at the recommended age should be given at any subsequent visit when indicated and feasible. The diagonally striped boxes indicate catch-up vaccination for age groups that warrant special effort to administer those vaccines not previously given. Additional vaccines may be licensed and recommended during the year. Licensed combination vaccines may be used whenever any components of the combination are indicated and the vaccine's other components are not contraindicated. Providers should consult the manufacturers' package inserts for detailed recommendations. *Extra hepatitis B vaccines in combination products may be given without harm if the combination product reduces the total number of vaccinations.* The American Academy of Pediatrics recommends a meningococcal vaccine prior to college or armed services entry.

NOTES

[1]*Hepatitis B vaccine* (HepB). All infants should receive the first dose of hepatitis B vaccine soon after birth and before hospital discharge; the first dose may also be given by age 2 months if the infant's mother is HBsAg-negative. Only monovalent HepB can be used for the birth dose. Monovalent or combination vaccine containing HepB may be used to complete the series. Four doses of vaccine may be administered when a birth dose is given. The second dose should be given at least 4 weeks after the first dose, except for combination vaccines, which cannot be administered before age 6 weeks. The third dose should be given at least 16 weeks after the first dose and at least 8 weeks after the second dose. The last dose in the vaccination series (third or fourth dose) should not be administered before age 6 months. Infants born to HBsAg-positive mothers should receive HepB and 0.5 mL hepatitis B immune globulin (HBIG) within 12 hours of birth at separate sites. The second dose is recommended at age 1–2 months. The last dose in the vaccination series should not be administered before age 6 months. These infants should be tested for HBsAg and anti-HBs at 9–15 months of age. Infants born to mothers whose HBsAg status is unknown should receive the first dose of the HepB series within 12 hours of birth. Maternal blood should be drawn as soon as possible to determine the mother's HBsAg status; if the HBsAg test is positive, the infant should receive HBIG as soon as possible (no later than age 1 week). The second dose is recommended at age 1–2 months. The last dose in the vaccination series should not be administered before age 6 months.

[2]*Diphtheria and tetanus toxoids and acellular pertussis vaccine* (DTaP). The fourth dose of DTaP may be administered as early as age 12 months, provided 6 months have elapsed since the third dose

and the child is unlikely to return at age 15–18 months. *Tetanus and diphtheria toxoids (Td)* vaccine is recommended at age 11–12 years if at least 5 years have elapsed since the last dose of tetanus and diphtheria toxoid–containing vaccine. Subsequent routine Td boosters are recommended every 10 years.

[3]*Haemophilus influenzae type b* (Hib) *conjugate vaccine*. Three Hib conjugate vaccines are licensed for infant use. If PRP-OMP (Pedvax-HIB or ComVax; Merck) is administered at ages 2 and 4 months, a dose at age 6 months is not required. DTaP/Hib combination products should not be used for primary immunization in infants at ages 2, 4, or 6 months, but can be used as boosters following any Hib vaccine.

[4]*Measles, mumps, and rubella vaccine* (MMR). The second dose of MMR is recommended routinely at age 4–6 years, but may be administered during any visit, provided at least 4 weeks have elapsed since the first dose and provided that both doses are administered beginning at or after age 12 months. Those who have not previously received the second dose should complete the schedule by the 11–12-year-old visit.

[5]*Varicella vaccine*. Varicella vaccine is recommended at any visit at or after age 12 months for susceptible children, i.e., those who lack a reliable history of chickenpox. Susceptible persons aged 13 years should receive two doses, given at least 4 weeks apart.

[6]*Pneumococcal vaccine*. The heptavalent *pneumococcal conjugate vaccine* (PCV) is recommended for all children age 2–23 months. It is also recommended for certain children age 24–59 months. *Pneumococcal polysaccharide vaccine* (PPV) is recommended in addition to PCV for certain high-risk groups. See *MMWR* 2000;49(RR-9);1–38.

[7]*Hepatitis A vaccine*. Hepatitis A vaccine is recommended for children and adolescents in selected states and regions and for certain high-risk groups; consult your local public health authority. Children and adolescents in these states, regions, and high-risk groups who have not been immunized against hepatitis A can begin the hepatitis A vaccination series during any visit. The two doses in the series should be administered at least 6 months apart. See *MMWR* 1999;48(RR-12); 1–37.

[8]*Influenza vaccine*. Influenza vaccine is recommended annually for children age 6 months with certain risk factors [including but not limited to asthma, cardiac disease, sickle cell disease, HIV, diabetes, and household members of persons in groups at high risk; see *MMWR* 2002;51(RR-3):1–31], and can be administered to all others wishing to obtain immunity. In addition, healthy children age 6–23 months are encouraged to receive influenza vaccine if feasible, because children in this age group are at substantially increased risk for influenza-related hospitalizations. Children aged 12 years should receive vaccine in a dosage appropriate for their age (0.25 mL if age 6–35 months or 0.5 mL if age 3 years). Children age 8 years who are receiving influenza vaccine for the first time should receive two doses separated by at least 4 weeks.

SUGGESTED READING

Centers for Disease Control and Prevention (CDC) Website. http://www.cdc.gov

CHAPTER 32
Fever in the Newborn
Gary A. Emmett

Although most babies with fever do not have sepsis, unfortunately, there is no perfect way to tell which children do have sepsis.

Fever promotes elimination of infection, but in the first few weeks of life fever also signals danger. Newborns do not have fully functional t-lymphocytes, which is why they contract yeast in the mouth and diaper areas so easily. Newborns also have passively acquired IgG that passes to the infant from its mother during gestation, particularly in the third trimester. Production of pyrogens, such as febrile agglutinins, is also limited. Therefore, fever in newborns is a relatively late sign in sepsis, because newborns have limited ability to respond to infection. In fact, the inability to maintain a normal temperature (being excessively high or low) is often the first sign in a newborn that the baby is infected.

"Fever" (why in quotation marks?—because in this case it is not necessarily a true fever, but only a temperature elevation from the environment) can also be passively acquired in a newborn. A mother with a fever will produce a newborn with a temporary elevation of temperature. If a newborn with a history of maternal temperature elevation is febrile on nursery admission and appears well, observe the newborn for several hours to see if the fever disappears. If the mother is diagnosed as having a uterine infection, the practitioner should obtain a blood culture from the baby and observe him or her. Many practitioners would also obtain a sterile urine culture and a complete blood count and may start antibiotics (See Chapter 9, GBS). In the same way, newborns can become warm from being overdressed and from elevated ambient temperature.

Why does the infant get warm or cold so quickly? The answer is found in the ratio of surface area to mass. An average (3.5 kg) newborn has more than three times the surface area per unit of mass as a 70-kg adult. Thus all forms of heat transfer (conduction, convection, radiation) have a magnified effect on newborns as compared to adults. A newborn also has a much larger percentage of that surface area in the head (about twice that of an adult). A hat is suggested until the newborn is completely temperature stable, which occurs when the child weighs 4 to 5 kg, has passed his or her due date, and is greater than a week old.

The hardest question to answer is what is a fever? Everyone agrees that 104°F (40°C) is a fever, but is 100.4°F (38°C) measured in the axilla a fever? How about 100.4°F (38°C) measured rectally? A temperature of 98.6°F (37°C) is "normal" temperature, because it is a whole number in the celsius measurement system that is near a human being's average temperature, not because everyone has that core temperature. The actual temperature of human beings varies by several degrees Fahrenheit during a 24-hour period, with the lowest measurement at about 0400 hours and the highest measurement late in the afternoon. Is 100.4°F (38°C) measured in the axilla a fever at 0400? Probably yes. Is 100.4°F (38°C) measured in the axilla a fever at 1600 hours? Maybe not.

The issue of where to measure the child's temperature is also controversial. Usually, but not always, the temperature of the forehead is less than the axilla, which is less than the mouth, which is less than the rectum. The standard place to measure the newborn temperature is the rectum, but rectal temperatures are not routinely done in many hospitals because of discomfort, embarrassment, and fear of litigation. Rectal temperatures are really quite safe if done properly—coat the thermometer tip with petroleum jelly or an equivalent lubricant, gently touch the center of the rectum, the rectum will "wink," and the thermometer can be gently slid in about 3 cm (1¹/₂ in.). The skin, axilla, and ear are the other frequent measurement sites. Studies showing the best method of measuring a temperature are quite confusing, but it is conclusive that the ear method is inconsistent in newborns because of the canal's small size.

Our advice for temperatures in the first 6 weeks of life:

- Use the axilla or the rectum to measure infant temperature.

- Measure until the temperature stops going up (check every 1 to 2 minutes).

- A temperature of 100.4°F (38°C) is a fever measured at any body site. An axillary temperature of 99.5°F (37.5°C) is suspicious and should be followed serially.

Table 32.1   Diagnosis and treatment of fever in children 28 days old and less

---

- *Blood culture*
- *Urine analysis and urine culture* obtained either by suprapubic aspiration or sterile catherization (see Table 32.2 for instructions)
- *CBC* with differential
- *Lumbar puncture* (see Table 32.3) with simultaneous *serum glucose*
- *Hospitalization and observation* until cultures are negative (at least 48 hr)
- *Treatment by parenteral antibiotics* that cover *E. coli, L. monocytogenes,* group B streptococci, and other gram-positive pathogens. Ampicillin and an aminoglycoside are commonly used. A third-generation cephalosporin is acceptable. (See Formulary, Appendix B, for dosages.)

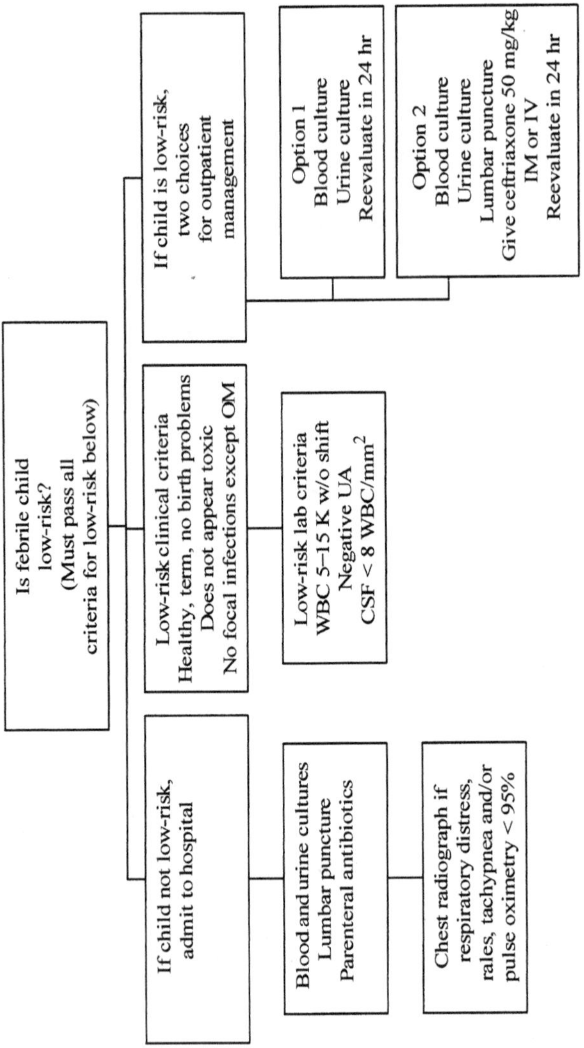

Is febrile child
low-risk?
(Must pass all
criteria for low-risk below)

Low-risk clinical criteria
Healthy, term, no birth problems
Does not appear toxic
No focal infections except OM

Low-risk lab criteria
WBC 5–15 K w/o shift
Negative UA
CSF < 8 WBC/mm^2

If child is low-risk,
two choices
for outpatient
management

Option 1
Blood culture
Urine culture
Reevaluate in 24 hr

Option 2
Blood culture
Urine culture
Lumbar puncture
Give ceftriaxone 50 mg/kg
IM or IV
Reevaluate in 24 hr

If child is not low-risk,
admit to hospital

Blood and urine cultures
Lumbar puncture
Parenteral antibiotics

Chest radiograph if
respiratory distress,
rales, tachypnea and/or
pulse oximetry < 95%

Figure 32.1　Sepsis workup for children 28–90 days old with fever.

Table 32.2   Sterile urethral catheterization

- Obtain sterile gloves, povidine iodine swabs, a 5 F sterile uréthral catheter, a package of sterile lubricant (such as K-Y Jelly), sterile fields, and a sterile urine cup. Procedure is most successful with an experienced second person to hold child in place and assist. Povidine iodine swabs, lubricant, and catheter must be opened and contents placed on a sterile field prior to procedure.
- By history, child should not have voided in the hour prior to the procedure.
- Place child on his/her back with assistant gently but firmly spreading legs by holding the thighs and knees.
- Clean with povidine iodine swabs three times, starting at urethra and cleaning in a spiral going outward, never inward, with each swab.
- Cover child's perineum with sterile field with central opening.
- Place one gloved hand to extend penis and retract foreskin (if present) or open labia. This hand is now not sterile. Place lubricated catheter in other gloved hand. Male urethra should be easily visualized. Female urethra is almost always directly anterior to the vagina. Insert the catheter gently, because one can easily make a false lumen. Slowly advance catheter until resistance is felt (the external sphincter), then increase pressure until catheter is easily advanced. Female bladder is within 5 cm of external sphincter; male bladder is within 5 cm plus the length of the penis. Collect urine in sterile cup (many practitioners place the distal end of the catheter in the sterile cup prior to insertion).
- Examining an unspun aliquot of the urine for white cells and bacteria is best, but requires experience. A dipstick for white cells and nitrates may substitute. *Unlike in adults and older children, in febrile children under 90 days, the urine culture is processed even if the dipstick is negative for WBCs and nitrate.*

Antipyretics (acetaminophen or ibuprofen) are not recommended for fever in very young children, because fever is taken so seriously (see the next paragraph). They are, however, recommended in procedural pain; see the Formulary in Appendix B.

The diagnostic workup of fever in children who are 28 days old or less is quite extensive. In various clinical studies, 60% to 80% of febrile children less than 90 days old had discernible causes of their fever such as otitis media, but at least 20% had no obvious cause of their fever. Studies show that the higher the fever, especially above 103°F (39.4°C), the higher the rate of occult bacteremia. Even a well-appearing child less than 90 days old with a fever of 103°F has a 3% chance of occult bacteremia, and therefore, a good chance to develop invasive disease

177

Table 32.3   Lumbar puncture

- *Is increased intracranial pressure present*? If so, image brain prior to lumbar puncture to prevent herniation.
- *Are platelets <50,000*? Is there a history of bleeding problems in child or family? Is skin infected in area of insertion? All these are contraindications for lumbar puncture.
- Place all needed equipment including four sterile specimen tubes on the sterile field.
- Draw an imaginary line between the iliac crests. The intervertebral space at or just caudal to this line is L3-4. Make an indelible mark on the skin at this point.
- An experienced assistant is essential. The plane of the child's back must be kept perpendicular to the table.
- Sit child up or lay on side with assistant holding the child's knees, hips, and neck flexed.
- Clean with povidine iodine swabs three times, starting at L-3 or L-4 and cleaning in a spiral going outward, never inward, with each swab.
- 0.5 to 1.0 cc of 1% lidocaine may be injected around insertion site, but it may make the site more difficult to use and is not used in many neonates.
- Using a $1^{1}/_{2}$-in. 21- to 23-gauge spinal needle with stylet, place tip just below spinal process and insert precisely in the midline aimed toward the umbilicus. The pop felt in older individuals is rare in the newborn. When spinal fluid starts to flow, obtain four specimen tubes. Measuring the opening pressure is almost never done in a child under 90 days.
- Obtain specimens for:
   CSF glucose and protein, and serum glucose. The glucose should be obtained simultaneously. The CSF glucose should be >2/3 of the serum glucose.
   Protein, which should be <100 mg/dL if tap is not bloody. (Also see Appendix A for assessing results.)
   Cell count and morphology: CSF cell count should be <10.
   Bacterial culture
   Herpes simplex (and other viruses if appropriate), PCR or culture.

such as pyelonephritis, osteomyelitis, or meningitis. A child under 90 days with elevation of the white cell count in the blood above 15,000 combined with a 104°F (40°C) or higher temperature may have as high as a 15% chance of occult bacteremia. Also, a white count below 5,000 may be a sign of overwhelming sepsis. Table 32.1 shows the minimal work up for a child 28 days and younger. For 29 days and older, see Fig. 32.1. Table 32.2 lists the steps for sterile urethral catheterization, and Table 32.3 lists considerations and procedures for lumbar puncture.

SUGGESTED READING

Burg FD, Ingelfinger JR, Polin RA, and Gershon A, (Eds.). *Gellis and Kagan's current pediatric therapy,* 17th ed. Philadelphia: WB Saunders, 2002.

CHAPTER 33

Bilirubin Follow-up after Discharge from the Well Baby Nursery

Gary A. Emmett

Jaundice follow-up after newborn nursery discharge is, in general, disorganized and dangerous, both to the baby and to the practitioner.

After discharge, babies can become more jaundiced with both indirect hyperbilirubinemia and direct hyperbilirubinemia. Indirect bilirubin can cause brain damage, as discussed in Chapter 15.

INDIRECT HYPERBILIRUBINEMIA

While trying to follow postdischarge bilirubin levels, documentation can become extremely difficult. Why? Because the patients that a practitioner sees in the nursery are often not the ones that he or she will see as an outpatient. This is especially true if the well nursery is run by hospital practitioners who in general do not see outpatients. Other interferences with good management include the following:

- Almost all the follow-up is done by phone.

- The results may not come back to the hospital doctor, but to the primary care physician.

- The results may be called in to the physician on call, instead of to the physician who ordered the tests.

- There is no chart available to record the data.

- The surname of the baby often changes after discharge.

Table 33.1 presents an action plan for newborn bilirubin posthospital follow-up. After the paperwork has been organized to facilitate the best treatment of patients, then uniformity of action must be achieved by a practice consensus, so that the care of your patients is dependent on their degree of jaundice and not on who is on call. A model treatment plan for hyperbilirubinemia is presented in Table 33.2.

Three treatment modalities are available for hyperbilirubinemia. Phototherapy with the Wallaby blanket, which can be used in the home, provides a blue light directly against the infant's skin. This treatment is practical for mildly elevated bilirubins. Phototherapy using

Table 33.1   Action plan for newborn bilirubin posthospital follow-up

Problem	Action Plan
Disorganized record keeping	1. Have all personnel in your practice use a standard form that includes the baby's birth date and birth hospital to minimize confusion. 2. Maintain forms in single location.
Multiple practitioners receiving data	Have a single practitioner correlate posthospital bilirubins in any given period of time.
Inconsistent treatment	Have a uniform hyperbilirubinemia treatment plan for all members of practice.
Inconsistency of infant surnames	File all records by birth date and birth hospital.

high-intensity lamps, an inpatient treatment, changes bilirubin to photobilirubin. The baby should be undressed, with eyes covered, while under these lamps. The lights should never be more than 15 inches from the baby, and if the bilirubin begins to go up to rapidly, multiple lighting devices may be used at the same time (including placing a Wallaby blanket under the infant). It is important to remember that the amount of light (the flux) received by the baby is inversely proportional to the square of the distance. If the light is twice as far away

Table 33.2   Model treatment plan for posthospital hyperbilirubinemia

1. Only fractionated infant bilirubins will be ordered for follow-up.
2. All outpatient infants with bilirubins designated as meriting follow-up by Table 15.4 will be retested every 24 to 48 hr until the total bilirubin has begun to drop.
3. All infants with elevated bilirubins should be kept in sunlight through the window as much as possible and should be fed every 2 to 3 hr.
4. An infant with a bilirubin between 16 and 18 mg/dL should be considered for home phototherapy.
5. An infant with a bilirubin of 18 mg/dL or greater should be admitted to the hospital, treated, and retested every 8–12 hr.

as indicated, the baby gets one quarter of the phototheraphy needed. Finally, for indirect bilirubins of greater than 20 mg/dL, the exchange transfusion is available. In the current era in the United States, these procedures should be referred to a neonatologist.

DIRECT HYPERBILIRUBINEMIA

Care for persistent direct bilrubin (the direct fraction is greater than 15% of the total bilirubin, and the bilirubin is significantly elevated for the child's age) is described in Chapter 13. The causes are listed in Table 13.1.

CHAPTER 34
Feeding and Feeding Problems
John Olsson

This issue generates more office calls than any other in the first few weeks of life.

As soon after delivery as possible, the newborn infant should be put to the breast. *Breast-feeding* should be encouraged whenever the infant is awake and interested in sucking, rather than on the nursery schedule. Initially, only a small amount of colostrum is available, but healthy term newborns require no supplementation, neither water nor formula.

The mother should drink one more quart (liter) of liquid each day than she did before her pregnancy. We also recommend she take an adult multivitamin with iron. If the mother has anxiety or technical problems with breast-feeding, peer or professional breast milk counselors can often alleviate the mother's anxieties. Rooming-in will enhance the mother's ability to provide all of her infant's feedings, as well as the rest of baby care.

Helping the mother learn proper feeding techniques is crucial. Proper positioning can usually prevent difficulty suckling and painful nipples. The infant is supported by the mother's arm with the infant's head elevated to the level of the nipple. The mother's other hand supports the breast and can introduce the nipple and areola into the infant's mouth. The infant's mouth must be open wide enough to close around the areola rather than latching onto the nipple itself. Attempts should be made to have the infant breast-feed from both breasts at each feeding, alternating the side the infant first latches on with each feeding. The infant should be burped after the first side, which helps stimulate the infant to nurse on the other side.

Milk production sufficient to cause breast enlargement usually takes 3 days to occur with a first-born infant, and may occur earlier with infants born to multiparous women. Once milk production has been established, the infant should be encouraged to feed every 2 to 3 hours, ideally emptying both breasts each time. Generally, when milk comes in, the infant stools with almost every feeding. The stool changes from dark green meconium to a yellow, seedy stool.

Inadequate breast-feeding can be avoided by encouraging mothers to breast-feed exclusively, frequently, and with proper technique. It is also helpful to decrease maternal stress by encouraging rest as well as adequate fluid and nutritional intake, while at the same time discouraging excessive visitation and social demands.

After discharge from the nursery, the physician or nurse clinician should see the breast-feeding infant for follow-up within the first week. The purpose of this visit is to assess how breast-feeding is going and whether there are problems that need to be addressed. Figure 34.1 shows pathways for inadequate feeding.

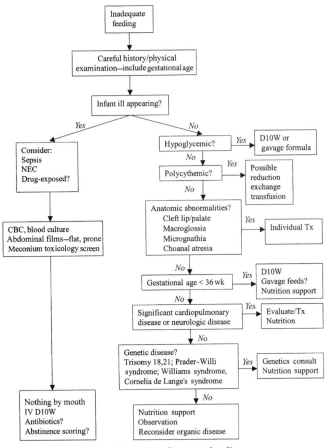

Figure 34.1   Inadequate feeding.

As soon as the infant has transitioned from delivery, having established a normal respiratory pattern and normal thermoregulation, and having demonstrated normal neurological activity, the infant who is going to be *bottle-fed* should be offered formula. Initial feeding with water or glucose-water is strongly discouraged. Formula provides more carbohydrates, helping the infant maintain normal glucose homeostasis. The danger of aspiration of the initial feed is equally low on water and formula. Various formulas are listed in Table 34.1.

Proper feeding technique with bottle-feeding involves the mother holding the infant in a position with the head above the rest of the body. It is not appropriate for the mother to feed the baby while the infant

Table 34.1   Selection of formulas and indication to use

Product Name	Indication to Use
Preterm human milk, mature human milk	Preterm infants will need human milk fortifier to support the needs of the growing premature infant. Mature human milk is ideal for growing term infants.
Enfamil human milk fortifier (HMF), Similac human milk fortifier	Human milk fortifiers are needed for low birth weight premature infants receiving breast milk. One packet HMF/25 mL breast milk makes 24 kcal/oz, and should be continued at least until 2000 g. Infants with BPD or congenital heart disease requiring fluid restriction may benefit beyond 2000 g.
Enfamil Premature formula, Similac Special Care. Both formulas are available in 20 kcal/oz and 24 kcal/oz.	For low birth weight premature infants. Continue these formulas at least until 2000 g. Infants with BPD or metabolic disease may benefit beyond 2000 g. Recommended continuing until 3.0–3.5 kg.
Similac Neosure, Enfacare	These discharge formulas provide preterm infants a nutrient intake that is between a preterm and term formula. Preterm infants can be transitioned to these formulas around 2000 g. The use of preterm discharge formulas to a postnatal age of 9 mo results in greater linear growth, weight gain, and BMC compared with the use of term formula (AAP).
Enfamil with iron (replaced in the U.S. by Enfamil Lipil), Gerber baby formula, Good Start, Lactofree, Similac with iron (replaced in U.S. by Similac Advance). For babies 0–12 mo.	Formulas for term infants. Available in ready-to-feed, powder, and liquid concentrate form. AAP recommends all formulas fed to infants be fortified with iron. Lactofree contains no lactose, but is not recommended for galactosemia.

(continued)

185

Table 34.1   (*Continued*)

Product Name	Indication to Use
Alsoy, Isomil (now in U.S. Isomil Advance), Gerber Soy, Isomil-SF, Isomil-DF, Prosobee (Now in U.S. Prosobee Lipil).	Feeding for term infants with galactosemia, hereditary lactase deficiency, documented transient lactase deficiency, or parents seeking vegetarian diets, documented IgE-mediated allergy to cow's milk. Soy formula is not recommended for birth weight <1800 g as per AAP.
Alimentum, Nutramigen, Pregestimil, Neocate	Hypoallergenic formulas for infants who are intolerant to intact proteins and with significant malabsorption due to gastrointestinal or hepatobiliary disease. Neocate is an elemental formula for infants intolerant to intact proteins and hydrolysates and can be used with infants after gut resection.
Portagen, Similac PM 60/40	Portagen is used in infants when long-chain triglycerides are poorly tolerated as in chylothorax or chylous ascites. Similac PM 60/40 with low minerals, low iron, and low renal solute formula is formulated for infants with renal problems and for any infants requiring low mineral infant formula.

is lying on the bed or in its bassinet. Initial feedings should contain a standard cow's milk formula with iron. Usually, initial feedings consist of 15 to 30 mL of formula given every 3 to 5 hours on demand. When feedings at this volume are tolerated, the volume may be advanced as the infant tolerates, with a goal of providing approximately 120 kcal/kg/day by the fifth day of life. As the volume increases, it is important that the parent burp the infant after every 1 to 2 oz to reduce the possibility of regurgitation.

Once an appropriate feeding pattern has been established, bottle-fed infants will usually void three to six times a day and stool with almost every feeding. The stools change from dark green meconium to a yellow, seedy stool.

It is unusual to have to change formulas for infants who are bottle-feeding. Regurgitation is frequently seen in the first few days of bottle-feeding and does not require a change in formula. Parents should be reassured, and one should be sure that the infant is being burped sufficiently. A family history of lactose intolerance or milk protein allergy warrants, especially when the infant is actually vomiting, a change of formula to an appropriate lactose-free formula or protein hydrolysate formula as indicated. Changing formulas from one cow's milk formula to another brand of cow's milk formula is not prudent.

Inadequate bottle-feeding is more frequently seen in more premature infants who may recover in the newborn nursery. These infants should have their caloric expectations calculated based on their birth weight. These infants may require gavage feedings if they are unable to achieve their fluid requirements. Premature infants may require formulas with increased caloric densities designed to meet their unique needs. Inadequate bottle-feeding can be avoided by encouraging the mother to provide all of her infant's feedings.

Inadequate feeding is defined as the insufficient intake of feeds due to an infant's inadequate oral motor skills or the infant's inability to sustain normal feeding effort. Generally, inadequate feeding affects hydration and/or nutritional status by the third to fifth day of life. Most infants are taking at least 100 kcal/kg/day by the fifth day of life. Inadequate feeding may be present from birth, or it may occur later in the perinatal period.

The history should include routine newborn history as well as feeding history. Complications of pregnancy, maternal medications during and following delivery, a history of illicit drug use or its risk factors, gestational age determinations, Apgar scores/resuscitation requirements, and sepsis risk factors are all important in the evaluation of the infant who does not feed well. It is important to determine if the infant who feeds poorly has always fed poorly or if the change in feeding has occurred quite suddenly. Sudden deterioration in feeding ability is more likely associated with sepsis, necrotizing enterocolitis (NEC), or a toxic/metabolic condition. The method of feeding, bottle versus breast, including the technique involved in either type of feeding, should be assessed. Stool frequency is often a better indicator of intake and is valuable in assessing inadequate feeding.

Physical examination should assist one in determining possible toxicity and overall cardiorespiratory stability. An ill-appearing infant may be septic or may have NEC. These infants must be made "nothing by mouth" (NPO) and evaluated urgently with laboratory tests and radiographs. Antibiotic therapy pending results of the sepsis evaluation is recommended. Drug-exposed infants may present as ill appearing, having hyperpyrexia, tachypnea, jitteriness, irritability, uncoordinated sucking, and vomiting. Significant cardiac or pulmonary disease should be identified and treated appropriately.

The infant who otherwise is not acutely ill may be evaluated systematically. Checking the serum glucose and hemoglobin is easy and may often be rapidly performed in the nursery environment. If these are abnormal, appropriate therapeutic interventions are indicated.

A thorough general examination (see Chapter 16) should identify anatomic abnormalities, including stigmata of genetic disease. A careful neurological examination will help identify those infants with a neuromuscular disease or the infant who has experienced birth asphyxia/birth trauma. One should assess the infant's overall tone, deep tendon and primitive reflexes, limb movement, sensation, and level of alertness.

One should confirm gestational age by a Ballard/Dubowitz examination. (See Chapter 17.) Feeding difficulty is common in premature and near-term infants. The collaboration of a multidisciplinary feeding team may be helpful in the infant's transition from gavage feeding to nipple feeding. If neurological injury is suspected, a premature infant may be evaluated using cranial ultrasound to evaluate for a possible intraventricular hemorrhage (IVH), and in term infants, a noncontrast computed tomography (CT) scan of the head may be considered to evaluate for subdural hemorrhage.

When the etiology remains unclear, one should support the infant nutritionally, observe, and reconsider possible organic etiologies for the poor feeding. Consultation with occupational and speech therapists experienced in infant feeding disorders may be helpful in assessing oral motor skills.

The history in a *vomiting* child should include routine newborn history as well as history specific to the assessment of emesis. See Fig. 34.2. Complications of pregnancy, labor, and delivery, including issues of gestational age and sepsis risk, are important. One should determine the time of onset of vomiting, frequency of vomiting, and the character of the vomiting process. It is useful to know what is contained in the emesis—that is, blood, mucus, or bile. It is also important to know how the infant is fed: Is the infant breast-feeding or bottle-feeding, what is the volume and type of formula, and what is the technique used in feeding or formula preparation? The presence or absence of stooling may be important if obstruction is being considered.

Physical examination should first involve assessing the infant for cardiorespiratory stability. Adequate hydration and stability of the circulation should be established. Inspection of the abdomen might disclose distension, a scaphoid quality, or abdominal wall erythema. Palpation will identify masses or organomegaly.

One of the first considerations will be to decide if an infant is actually vomiting, or simply regurgitating, or "spitting." Vomiting is forceful and often preceded by nausea or retching. Regurgitation is a passive movement of stomach contents into the esophagus. Regurgitation is rarely serious or an obstacle to appropriate weight gain, whereas vomiting may be life threatening.

Bilious vomiting is an emergency in the infant of any age. It often suggests an underlying surgical condition warranting prompt evaluation and treatment. Malrotation, with or without volvulus, may be suggested by findings of obstruction on a abdominal radiograph. NEC should be considered in a premature infant who presents with abdominal distention, bilious vomiting, and blood in the stools. As many as

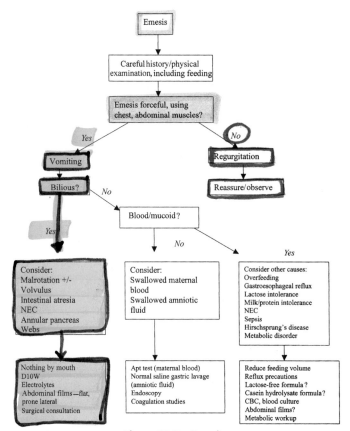

Figure 34.2   Emesis.

35% of cases of NEC may occur in full-term newborns. Early bilious vomiting may occur in the setting of intestinal atresia, though more distal atresias/stenoses may present later in the neonatal course. Meconium ileus may present as a case of small bowel obstruction. Hirschsprung's disease usually will present later, often associated with delayed or infrequent stooling.

Mucoid or mucoid and blood-mixed emesis is not uncommon. The infant may swallow maternal blood and amniotic fluid in the course of delivery. Ingesting maternal blood during breast-feeding through cracked maternal nipples is also not infrequent. One may differentiate maternal blood from infant blood by performing an Apt test. Ingestion of mucoid amniotic fluid may cause emesis and may be treated

189

with gastric lavage with 30 to 60 mL of normal saline until clear. More serious bleeding warrants evaluation of the infant's coagulation process. Rarely, endoscopy may also be required to evaluate upper gastrointestinal bleeding. Other causes to consider should include overfeeding, gastroesophageal reflux, formula intolerance, and sepsis.

SUGGESTED READING

Websites are very good sources for nutrition information, and because the composition of formulas is constantly changing, more up-to-date than many texts.
KidsHealth: http://www.kidshealth.org/
Nutrition and Your Child: http://www.bcm.tmc.edu/cnrc/consumer/nyc/nyc.htm
U.S. Maternal and Child Health Bureau: http://www.mchb.hrsa.gov/default.htm

CHAPTER 35
Breathing Difficulties
Gary A. Emmett

People are always very concerned about how their babies breathe. Mothers lie awake at night just assuring themselves that their child is still audibly breathing. Here are some ideas to help you reassure the new mother, and yourself, that everything is fine.

The best way to discover the cause of noisy or inefficient breathing in a patient is by approaching it logically.

Step 1—Is the abnormal sound physiologically significant?

If the child is eating and gaining weight (minimal weight gain for a newborn is 15 g per day), if the baby can sleep for at least an hour after feedings, and if the baby is happy and playful, the unusual breathing sound is not clinically significant, and the cause does not have to be pursued.

Step 2—Is the problem inspiratory or expiratory?

When parents worry about their child's breathing, answering this question is a good place to start in discovering a pathologic origin of the child's symptoms. In general, inspiratory difficulties involve the upper airway, whereas expiratory problems involve the lungs. Causes of upper airway obstruction in the newborn are listed in Table 35.1. Causes of lower airway obstruction in the newborn are listed in Table 35.2.

Step 3—Does the child have signs of respiratory distress?

Table 35.3 lists the signs of respiratory distress in a newborn. Many babies will have a single one of these four symptoms at times without underlying pathology.

Just after birth and during the first 24 hours of life, many babies have what is called transient tachypnea of the newborn (TTN). This condition, much more common after Caesarean delivery, is caused by inadequate squeezing of the fluid out of the walls of the lungs by the delivery process. These children, though often extremely tachypnic, are not in significant distress at any time and do not look ill. Respiratory rates of 90 for a few hours are not uncommon. For details of treatment for infants in respiratory distress, see Chapter 6.

Step 4—Is the child apneic?

Normal infantile respiration is rhythmically arrhythmic. Infants normally breathe in bursts, with no breathing for 5 to 8 seconds followed by many short breaths. Sometimes the pattern is beyond the acceptable

Table 35.1   Causes of upper airway obstruction

Disease	Symptom	Diagnostic Method
Choanal atresia/stenosis	Child opens mouth to breathe	Pass a wet 8 F feeding tube through each naris to the pharynx
Epiglottis	Drooling	Lateral neck X-ray
Paralyzed vocal chord(s)	Patient very hoarse	Observe with direct laryngoscopy
Croup	Much worse at night	History/stethoscope
Mass impinging on trachea: Hemangioma Aberrant blood vessel Benign tumor	Worsens with time	Flexible laryngoscope
Tracheamalacia	Varying degrees of stridor	Barium swallow/ flexible laryngoscope
Tracheoesphageal fistula	Frequent pneumonia	Barium swallow/ flexible laryngoscope
Foreign body above trachael bifurcation (iatrogenic)	Whistling	X-ray of upper airway

Table 35.2   Causes of lower airway obstruction

Disease	Symptom	Diagnostic Method
Aspiration	Meconium beyond vocal chords at birth	Chest X-ray (CXR)
Congestive heart failure	Fine rales/dependent edema	CXR/echocardiogram
Pneumothorax	Crepitious under skin	CXR
Pneumonia	Wet cough	CXR
Myocarditis/ pericarditis	Tachycardia	Echocardiogram
Foreign body in lungs (iatrogenic)	Whistling/unequal breath sounds	CXR

Table 35.3   Objective measures of respiratory distress in an infant

- Tachypnea: Respiratory rate consistently above 50 breaths per min
- Nasal flaring
- Retraction of the rib cage and abdomen with breathing
- Cyanosis of the face or body at any time (the hands of a cold child are usually cyanotic and not a good diagnostic sign of respiratory distress)
- Pulse oximetry should be greater than 95%

Table 35.4   Causes of apnea

- Obstructive apnea: Any of the processes in Table 35.1 can lead to problems completely expanding the lungs. Eventually, this may lead to apnea and then cyanosis, brain damage, and eventually death. Many adults and older children have sleep apnea, which is the same process.
- Intrinsic apnea: On some occasions, apnea is caused by an inability of the respiratory center in the midbrain to function properly. Preterm infants and infants with severe neurological damage are often apneic. Occasionally, full-term babies who are otherwise normal will become apneic. The premature and full-term babies who are otherwise neurologically intact will grow out of this apnea in about two months to a year.
- Infectious apnea: Many respiratory infections of young infants are associated with apnea and sometimes death. Respiratory syncytial virus (RSV), pertussis, and adenovirus are common childhood infections associated with apnea in young children.

norm. Periods of apnea should not exceed 15 seconds. Some physicians believe that infantile apnea is a major cause of sudden infant death syndrome (SIDS). Table 35.4 lists causes of apnea. A pneumogram done with a four-channel thermistor is the most reliable test on whether apnea is obstructive or intrinsic.

SUGGESTED READING

American Academy of Pediatrics contributors and reviewers. International Guidelines for Neonatal Resuscitation: an excerpt from the Guidelines 2000 for Cardiopulmonary Resuscitation and Emergency Cardiovascular Care: International Consensus on Science. *Pediatrics* 2000;106:E29.

CHAPTER 36

Urination and Defecation

Gary A. Emmett

Parents are obsessed with their child's elimination patterns. Thorough knowledge of the acceptable limits of normal will enable the practitioner to comfort many a parent.

URINATION

The average child, after the first few days of life, will need between 120 and 180 mL per kg per day of liquids. How often a child urinates is dependant on many factors, including the child's own physiology and the amount of moisture in the child's environment. The minimum urination in a 24-hour period for an infant is three thoroughly soaked diapers. Of course, a child can have many more. If a child appears to be drinking sufficient amounts and yet not urinating with the frequency or amount that one expects, then the environmental and physiological factors listed in Table 36.1 should be considered.

Infants can also get too dry because they urinate too frequently. The only common causes of this problem are diabetes and the syndrome of inappropriate antidiuretic hormone (SIADH). Diabetes in infants is often caused by general pancreatic failure rather than classic type one diabetes, but either is possible.

DEFECATION

Both constipation and diarrhea are common in the first few weeks of life. To many lay people, the definitions of these conditions are very unclear. When parents tell you that their child has diarrhea or constipation, the first question is, "What do you mean by that?" Constipation and diarrhea are defined in Table 36.2.

A proper history includes actual numbers of stools a day and the color and consistency of each one. Very commonly, a parent will tell the pediatric practitioner that a child has constipation because it strains when it has a bowel movement. Infants normally strain when they have bowel movements. Sitting the infant up will often minimize the straining by having gravity assist the defecation.

Constipation is rarely caused by disease, but is common in children with cystic fibrosis, Hirschsprung's disease, and obstruction and narrowing of the gastrointestinal tract. The most common cause of constipation is simply not getting enough free fluid in the child's diet. Treat hard, painful stooling with sugar water (one tablespoon of granular

Table 36.1   Causes of less than optimal urination

Environmental
- Overly dry ambient air—mechanically heating or cooling the air markedly reduces its humidity. A well-sealed house on a cold January day heated up to 73°F will have a humidity of 11% or 12%, which is less than the average humidity in the Mohave Desert.
- Overly absorbent diapers—some new disposable diapers absorb water so well, it is difficult to determine whether they are wet or not. It is better to judge whether a diaper is soaked by its weight rather than by its apparent moisture.

Physiological
- Obstruction of the urinary tract—the most common cause is posterior urethral valves. Valves causing partial closure may not show up until the child is 1 or 2 weeks old. A child with a physical obstruction of the urinary tract is in pain and is very irritable.
- Kidney failure—the average creatinine for a child is 0.1 mg/dL per year. Infants rarely have creatinines greater than 0.3 mg/dL.
- Urinary tract infection—children in urinary pain may not urinate.

sugar or Karo syrup in 4 oz of water), giving a minimum of 2 oz twice a day. Or give diluted all-natural adult noncitrus juice, specifically apple, grape, and prune; mix 2 oz of water with 2 oz of pure juice, and give 2 to 4 oz of the mixture daily.

Diarrhea can be caused by metabolic disorders such as chloride loosing diarrhea syndrome or by poor absorption of the diet. Poor absorption results from intolerance of proteins found in the milk. Changing formula to a non-lactose-containing formula for bottle-fed babies, and minimizing laxatives, fruit juices, and whole grain products in the mother's

Table 36.2   Definitions

Constipation	Hard, rocklike stools at any time *or* stools that occur less often than every 72 hr in a bottle-fed baby and less often than every 96 hr in a breast-fed baby.
Diarrhea	Bottle-fed babies with stools that lack consistency or occur more than six times in a 24-hr period during the first month of life or more than four times in a 24-hr period after the first month of life. Breast-fed babies with stools that have no solid portion at all and occur more than six times in a 24-hr period.

Note: Odiferous stools imply incomplete absorption and are usually related to the formula and not to the baby's physiology.

195

diet for breast-fed babies, may ameliorate chronic diarrhea. Using electrolyte solutions or no food by mouth orders to reduce diarrhea in infants is dangerous and should not be tried outside of the hospital setting.

OTHER ABNORMALITIES OF THE GI TRACT

Spitting up blood or having blood in the bowel movement of a new infant may be protein intolerance (either cow's milk or mother's), or may simply be swallowed blood if mother is breast-feeding and her breasts are sore. Infected milk glands often secrete significant amounts of blood.

Acolic stools (pale to white) are a sign of liver malfunction, and if persistent more than 24 hours, should be followed up by liver enzyme studies.

Often parents come in worried their child is urinating blood. If they present a diaper with a violently pink color where the urine was deposited, this is simply uric acid crystals with a pink to orange color and has no clinical significance.

SUGGESTED READING

KidsHealth. www.kidshealth.org (2003).

C H A P T E R 37

Dermatology

Linda Meloy

Skin lesions in the newborn can easily baffle the newcomer. Dr. Meloy attempts to give a systematic approach to dissipate the confusion.

In newborns, skin lesions that appear pathologic can often have no long-term significance (such as nevus flammeus), or those that appear innocuous may be a sign of serious disease (such as café au lait spots).

Start by simply categorizing the lesion as in Fig. 37.1. After the lesion is characterized as a macule, papule, vesicle, and so forth, then go through the individual algorithms to identify the appropriate newborn lesion.

Papular/macular rashes have many origins and levels of morbidity (see Fig. 37.2). *Erythema toxicum,* which is a wheal with a red base around a central white papule, is allergic in nature, is transitory (comes and goes within hours), and is caused by eosinphils secreting IgE (Fig. 37.3). It is innocuous, can be seen within a few hours of birth, and can continue for up to 6 weeks.

Contact dermatitis, a rough-to-touch erythema that blanches with pressure, can be treated by removing the offending surface (often bed-clothes) or may need 1% hydrocortisone twice a day for 5 to 7 days if it persists.

Milia, which are white, smooth-to-touch papules, usually on the face (Fig. 37.4), will spontaneously resolve by 3 months and are superficial inclusion cysts of the skin related to Epstein's pearls in the mouth. They differ from neonatal acne, which is a *P. acnes*–infected sebaceous follicle identical in pathology to adolescent acne. Both milia and acne usually disappear by 3 months. If acne persists past 3 months, obtaining a testosterone level may be in order.

Candida dermatitis (Fig. 37.5), which has red satellites, is found most often in the mouth (thrush) and perianally. Antifungal topical medication may be required for resolution, such as nystatin oral suspension for thrush (2 cc rubbed around infant's mouth and, if breast-feeding, the mother's nipples) or nystatin cream three times a day to diaper area for diaper dermatitis.

Streptococcus A cellulitis, which is red, warm, tender, and does not blanch, requires antibiotic therapy. *Miliaria crystallina* occurs in warm areas and consists of raised fine papules. Treatment includes not over-dressing the infant and cooling the child's room.

Neonatal lupus is associated with maternal lupus, usually ssA(Ro) and ssB(La). The clinician should be alert for heart block and thrombocytemia, which also occur. If the rash persists, often steroids are

Macules
Papules

Vesicles
Pustules

Petechiae

Pigmented
Lesions

Hemangiomas

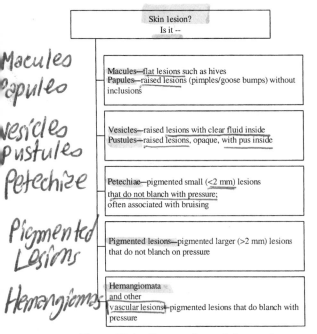

Figure 37.1   Dermatology of the newborn.

required. *Congenital rubella*, with its flushed facial rash and adenopathy, is very rare in the United States, but 5 or more cases occur annually, especially to new immigrants.

When vesicles and/or pustules lesion are present, the lesion may be cultured for infection and treated. See Fig. 37.6. Neonatal infections with these organisms can be life threatening, and treatment is emergent.

Staphylococcus aureus (Fig. 37.7) is the most common cause of pathologic bacterial infections of the skin. These pustular lesions become crusty with a gold-colored scab (Fig. 37.8) as they open up, and are found in skin folds, especially around the umbilicus in the first few weeks of life. These require antibiotics, intravenously if ill. Cultures of blood and the local site are strongly recommended. For a single isolated lesion in a child who is afebrile, mupirocin cream (Bactroban) applied three times a day is adequate. For an afebrile child with periumbilical erythema and pustulant discharge, oral cephalexin, 15 mg per kg per dose three times daily, is acceptable in a well child with a negative blood culture. Any fever in an infant or lesions in multiple locations requires an inpatient course.

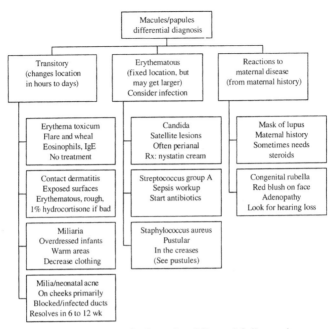

Figure 37.2   Macules/papules differential diagnosis.

Streptococcus group B and even group A may cause similar lesions. The lesions need to be cultured, a sepsis workup done, and parenteral antibiotics begun. A Tzanck smear may help identify *herpes lesions,* but will also be positive with varicella. Herpes lesions need to be cultured, and acyclovir at 60 mg per kg per day divided into three doses for 14 to 21 days can be given. In an infant, this course should start out as parenteral.

Varicella requires VZIG, vaccine, and 30 mg per kg per day of acyclovir in baby isolation. See Chapter 14 for details. *Cytomegalovirus* requires treating the retinitis with cidofovir 5 mg per kg one time given with probenecid and hydration then weekly maintenance with cidofovir 3 mg per kg again with probenecid and hydration.

Children with the genetic lesions of *ichthyosis, epidermal bullosis, incontinentia pigmenti,* and *ectodermal dysplasia* have many problems, but their prime acute care problem is infection. All these conditions promote invasive skin infection. The best way to attempt to stop sepsis is by providing artificial barriers with continuous moisturization with emollients and by aggressively treating any signs of infection, especially fever.

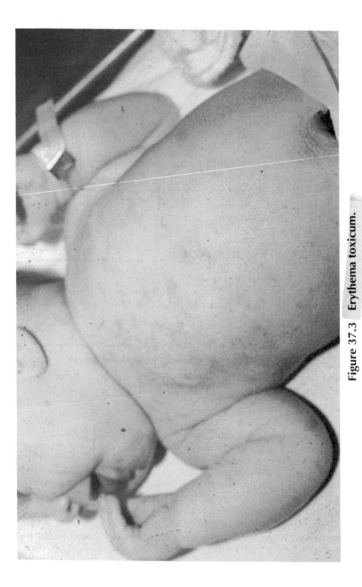

Figure 37.3 Erythema toxicum.

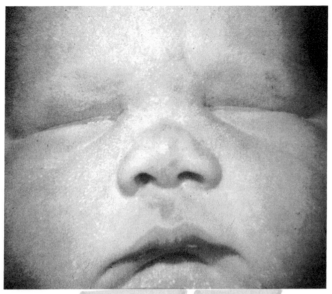

Figure 37.4   Milia on the chin and nevus flammeus on both eyelids.

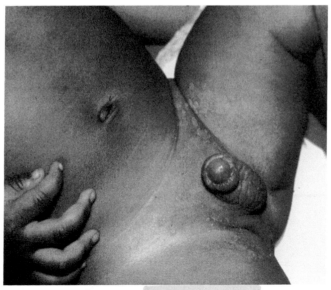

Figure 37.5   Candida dermatitis.

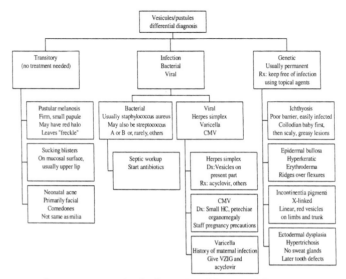

Figure 37.6   Vesicules/pustules differential diagnosis.

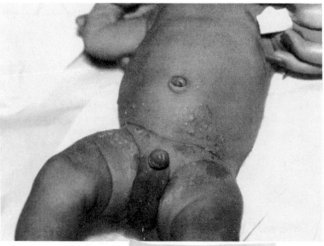

Figure 37.7   Staphylococcus infection.

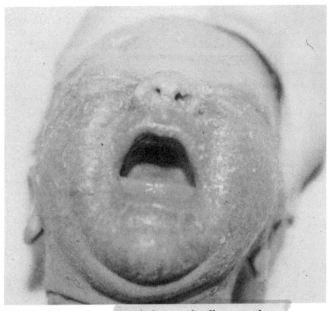

Figure 37.8 Staphylococcal yellow crusting.

Some very sinister-appearing lesions are quite innocuous and self-resolving. *Pustular melanosis* is probably viral and consists of off-white papules that contain small (less than 1 cc) waxy pellets. The lesions are in groups on flat surfaces and form in utero. When the papules open, "freckles" are permanently left on the skin.

Sucking blisters are large vesicles found on the mucosal surface of the lips, the skin around the mouth, the hands, and the arms. They appear to be "traction" lesions from simply sucking very hard. They appear to be painless and disappear with time. *Neonatal acne lesions* usually occur on the face. For details, see the paragraph on milia.

Ectodermal aplasia appears as denuded blister(s) with no dermis beneath when the blister resolves. The cause is unknown. If on the scalp (the most common location), no hair follicles form and there is lifelong local alopecia.

Petechiae can result from trauma, and a history and distribution appropriate to the lesion found confirms the origin. See Fig. 37.9. If the child has an abnormal neurological examination and a history of head trauma, imaging the head for intracranial bleeding is suggested. Ultrasound with a skillful operator is not invasive and requires no anesthesia. *Maternal thrombocytopenia* can lead to newborn thrombocytopenia, but infection must be considered.

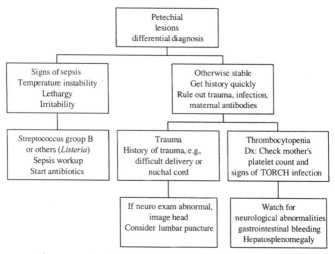

Figure 37.9   Petechial lesions differential diagnosis.

Infections such as *bacterial sepsis* (especially from listeria monocytogenes) produce petechiae. Any newborn who is not interacting well with the environment or has a fever or other physical signs of illness (such as nonresolving irritability) requires a sepsis workup (see Chapter 32) and is treated with ampicillin and an aminoglycoside.

Pigmented lesions are permanent, although they seem to lighten gradually with age in most cases. See Fig. 37.10. There are too many types to even list, but common ones include the following:

Mongolian spots are primarily gray-blue lesions, but have many colors depending on the depth of pigmentation in the epidermis and dermis. They are found in 95% of African Americans, 81% of Asian Orientals, 70% of Latinos, 62% of Asian Indians, and 10% of white infants. They are grossly symmetrical and almost always cover the buttocks.

Café au lait spots occur in approximately 20% of newborns, but may be associated with many syndromes, most prominently neurofibromatosis and McCune-Albright syndrome.

Darker lesions, the nevus of Ito and in the orbital area the nevus of Ota, are associated with glaucoma and require ophthalmologic exam. Hairy congenital nevi have a malignant potential and are often removed later in life. Sebaceous nevi are found on the scalp, are yellow-orange in color, and are devoid of hair. They are slightly raised and oily.

Figure 37.11 provides details about hemangiomas. Vascular *nevus flammeus simplex* or salmon patch are telangiectactic lesions, which blanch and are commonly on the neck, glabella, forehead, or upper lip. Many disappear by the child's first birthday, but neck and glabella lesions remain and increase with excitement.

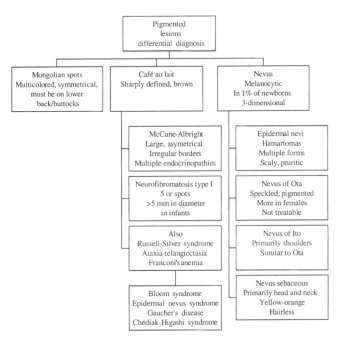

Figure 37.10   Pigmented lesions differential diagnosis.

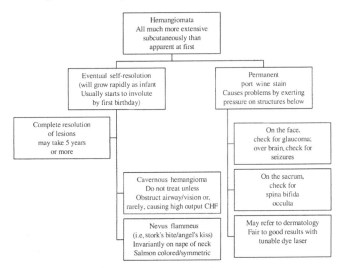

Figure 37.11   Hemangiomata.

205

Capillary hemangiomas blanch with pressure and grow faster than the infant. They involute with time, with significant regression by age 12 months and disappearance in most cases by age 5 years. Capillary hemangiomas may obstruct airways or trap platelets as in Kasabach-Merritt syndrome. Most capillary hemangiomas first grow with the child and then regress.

Port wine stains, which do not blanch, are not raised, and are darker than hemangiomas, are associated with glaucoma near the eye, brain vessel angiomatosis with seizures (Sturge-Weber syndrome), and spina occulta near the lumbar region. They cause disease by direct pressure on other structures. They may respond to laser surgery for cosmetic reasons.

SUGGESTED READING

American Academy of Pediatrics. *Red book 2003: report of the Committee on Infectious Diseases,* 26th ed. Elk Grove Village, IL: Author, 2000.

Fletcher MA. *Physical diagnosis in neonatology.* Philadelphia: Lippencott-Raven, 1998.

Johr R, Schachner L. Neonatal dermatological challenges. *Pediatr Rev* 1997;18:86–94.

Thureen P, ed. *Assessment and care of the well newborn.* Philadelphia: WB Saunders, 1999.

CHAPTER 38

High-Risk Newborn Follow-Up

William McNett

The rapid advancement in the therapy of high-risk newborns frequently brings to the general pediatrician graduates of the intensive care nursery who have many chronic conditions and multiple medications. This is a short guide on what to do about these nontraditional patients.

Providing general pediatric care to the intensive care nursery (ICN) graduate is challenging and frightening to the general pediatrician. The neonatologists have invested an enormous amount of both time and resources in the patient prior to the first visit to your office. The parents have been through an emotional and physically trying time during their infant's often turbulent stay in the ICN. The first office visit can be overwhelming for the parents, the practitioner, and the office staff:

- The parents consider this patient fragile (and will continue to worry for a long time) while they are struggling with the child's small size, often a large amount of medical equipment, and the child's complex care issues.

- The practitioner is bewildered by the chronicity and complexity of the care needed by these children, both of which are relatively rare issues in pediatrics.

- The staff may have to get multiple approvals from the insurers and give multiple referrals for all the specialist visits needed.

The only way to get everything right from the first visit on is to have a systematic approach that can be seen in Table 38.1.

For the medically complicated patient, the practitioner must create allies to supplement and enrich the care of these newborns. Most insurers have case management available, but the new high-risk infant may not have a case manager automatically assigned. The parents and/or the practitioner must request a case manager for any special-needs child. Most of these children have been evaluated by the neonatal intensivist and one or more pediatric specialists. Requests for records should be sent to each of these specialists and their opinions sought for short- and long-term follow-up. For any complex long-term issue, a specialist should be familiar with the problem and a care plan developed. If the

Table 38.1   Allies in high-risk neonate care

Allies	Function
Insurers' risk management	Authorizes and expedites availability of needed goods and services
Neonatalogist	Helps coordinate long-term care by defining ongoing problems and short-term goals
Pediatric specialists	Define treatment care plans for specific problems
Early intervention team	Has resources to provide long-term rehabilitation until child is of school age
Local rehabilitation therapists	Provide interim therapy until early intervention starts, and supplemental therapy if early intervention does not meet child's needs
Social workers	Coordinate and expedite multiple therapeutic care plans and act as child advocate for needed services

infant has developmental issues, the early intervention team (a federal mandate in the United States, but each team is organized and run locally) is a potent ally. Because it is often months before the early intervention team can rule on eligibility and institute therapy, early assessments by physical, occupational, and speech therapists may be solicited to evaluate and to start therapy as quickly as possible. The local rehabilitation specialists may also supplement the early intervention team's work if the child appears to need more intense therapy than is available by statute. Finally, a social worker or team can coordinate the different requests for home services, equipment, and nursing needs and expedite their availability. Social work is also an advocate for the patient when services seem inadequate for therapeutic needs.

Visit frequency for high-risk children is much more often than in most well baby care. Table 38.2 describes these follow-up visits. A patient must be seen frequently (at least every week) until the child achieves a steady weight gain, the parents are comfortable with their multitude of caregiving tasks, and none of the ICN follow-up issues are acute. The use of palivizumab (Synagis), which must be given monthly, also influences the next health maintenance visit along with the need to administer timely immunizations. See Table 38.3 provides further information.

High-risk newborns often need special formulae (see Tables 38.4 and 38.5). They also have chronic conditions that have special follow-up needs (see Table 38.6).

Table 38.5   Preparation of standard infant formula to increase caloric density

Formula Type	Caloric Concentration (kcal/oz)	Amount of Formula	Water (oz)
Liquid concentrate	20	13 oz	13 oz
	22	13 oz	10.5 oz
	24	13 oz	8.5 oz
	27	13 oz	6 oz
Powder formula	20	4 scoops	8 oz
(Rounded to the nearest 0.5 scoop)	22	4.5 scoops	8 oz
	24	5 scoops	8 oz
	27	5.5 scoops	8 oz

Table 38.6   Common diagnoses and their follow-up in high-risk neonates

Diagnosis	Treatment	Follow-up
Chronic lung disease (bronchopulmonary dysplasia)	• Diuretics • Bronchodilators • Oxygen • Hypercaloric formula (22–27 cal/oz)	• Follow respiratory rates • Pulse oximetry • Growth • Serum electrolytes depending on type of diuretic used
Retinopathy of prematurity	• Close observation • Laser surgery • Vitrectomy	• Serial exams by pediatric retinology Follow up at 6–12 mo (adjusted age) by a pediatric ophthalmologist
Necrotizing enterocolitis	• Surgical intervention • Delayed feeding/nutrition • Hydrolysate casein protein formula	• Observe for signs of abdominal obstruction due to adhesions

(continued)

Table 38.6   (*Continued*)

Diagnosis	Treatment	Follow-up
Apnea of prematurity	• Apnea monitor • Methylxanthine (caffeine, theophylline)	• Serial downloads of apnea monitor every 2–4 wk until normal • Monitor serum caffeine/theophylline levels
Gastroesophageal reflux	• Chalasia precautions (keep upright during and after feeds, thicken feeds with 1–3 tsp rice cereal per oz of formula, elevate head of crib) • Prokinetic agent • H2 antagonist • Gastric acid pump inhibitor • Antacid	• Follow for clinical signs • Follow growth • Adjust medications for weight • Generally resolves by 6–9 mo (adjusted age)
Intraventricular hemorrhage (grade III or IV)		• Serial head circumference • Developmental screens • Serial head ultrasound • Early intervention
Neonatal rickets	• Premature infant formula • Calcium supplement • Phosphorus supplement	• Alkaline phosphate level

SUGGESTED READING

The Medical Home site of the AAP is one of the best for the detailed follow-up of special babies—http://www.medicalhomeinfo.org/

CHAPTER 39

Talking to Parents

Budd N. Shenkin

This chapter will help you establish a caring connection with the baby and its family.

ESTABLISHING THE PATIENT-PRACTITIONER CONNECTION

All patients (patients meaning both the baby and the family) are different: some are suspicious from the start, some give you the benefit of the doubt, and some indulge their need to be cared for by immediately giving you a halo. But whatever the patients' tendency, to accept you as their caregiver, all patients need to believe that you possess three specific qualities:

- You care about the baby and its family.

- You are competent.

- You are reliable.

These are the three cardinal clinical virtues. If your patients believe you have these three qualities, they will stick with you through thick and thin. You will get the wish of most doctors—you will be appreciated.

The patient does not need to believe that you are perfect or that you never sleep. They should not expect you to get everything right all the time, because nobody does. But they need to feel that, because you care about them as people and because you take pride in your profession, you will do your very best. They will expect that:

- You will attempt to resolve all issues.

- You will be medically competent, but still practical.

- You will call for consultation, or transfer the baby appropriately, because you have the judgment not to go beyond your capabilities.

The best way of showing that you care is to be empathetic. In spite of sometimes adverse working conditions, one cannot lose the common feeling with patients, or an important part of medicine will be

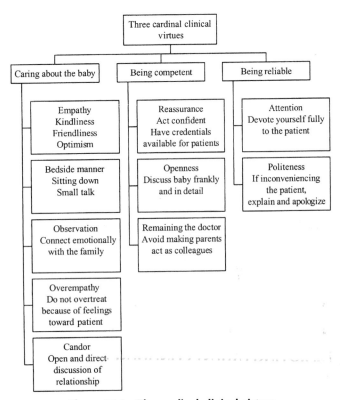

Figure 39.1   The cardinal clinical virtues

lost, the part that keeps you human and makes it worthwhile to be a doctor. Simply talking sympathetically with your patients can lead to a solution.

Express your empathy either overtly or subtly with every visit. Kindness, friendliness, and optimism go a long way, but openness is equally important. Sitting down for 30 seconds and chatting with the family conveys a feeling of caring and leisureliness. Small talk helps: it gives the impression of not letting a busy schedule interfere with the human interaction. Studies show that patients believe these actions are signs of a longer, more detailed visit. The extra time caring takes is negligible, and, in fact, you can save time because the family is usually less reticent to discuss emotion-laden issues.

Do not permit your caring to prevent close observation of the family. Are they responding to you as you would hope? Have you connected with the family? You may have failed to achieve a therapeutic alliance (where you and the family see yourselves on the same team). The family may want therapy or consultation that you believe is fruitless. Or it could be something less tangible; they appear not satisfied with you and your therapeutic course. If you find any of these things happening, you have a choice. Unfortunately, what most practitioners do is to soldier on, trying to maintain a positive attitude toward the family: acting kindly, answering factual questions semicompliantly, and maybe complaining about them to colleagues or nurses. These patients become the "difficult family."

There is, however, a better choice available: make a direct observation about the relationship between you and the patient. For instance, say to the patient, "Do you mind if I say something? I'm not sure we're communicating here as well as I would like to. You seem real anxious about things, and I can't seem to calm you down. And you seem to have a lot of questions about the care we are giving your baby. What do you think? Be honest. You and your baby come first."

After your candor, the conversation can go many ways. By confronting a troublesome relationship directly, by addressing the relationship itself, you stand a chance to make a direct improvement. If a poor patient-practitioner connection continues, suggest that the patient transfer to a colleague. Part of being a professional is realizing you cannot please everyone. Most of the time, if you allow your patients to be open, they will relax and an improved therapeutic relationship will occur.

IMPROVING PATIENT CONFIDENCE

Along with establishing a positive patient-practitioner connection, ensuring patient confidence is also crucial. Most patients assume that you know what you are doing. Patients often trust your institution or the obstetrician who referred them to you, but placing a minibiography of yourself in your newborn handout will reassure most patients about your credentials. Your manner counts—act as if you trust yourself, and that is how your patients will view you.

Keep the parents informed about the baby, especially if things are not going well. Reassure them—show the parents that you know how to deal with the situation. Tell them promptly when you need the help of a specialist or the baby needs to be transferred to a tertiary care institution. Discussing prognosis is always important. Patients trust a doctor with a road map. Do not go into obscure scientific minutia about the baby with the parents, but involving them in important therapeutic decisions empowers them. *Note: Do not forget to inform the obstetrician about the baby's course. A wise pediatrician is always kind to obstetricians.*

Many small gestures increase patient confidence in you:

• Practicing team medicine increases your reliability. (When you come in and are able to say, "Dr. Ryan told me all about you," your patients will feel more important.)

• If you are late or dealing with something else, you mention it, apologize for it, and then pay full attention to the patient.

AFTER CHILDBIRTH

Childbirth is a "happy trauma," both physically and emotionally. There can be a conflict of expectations and reality. Parents may feel that they are expected to be fairy-tale happy, in spite of sleep deprivation and many minor worries. Mothers may feel pressed to be perfect although their bodies ache and their hormones are awry. Fathers may feel pressure to be supportive, whereas what they really want is to be supported. Reassurance can be helpful. Caregivers need to know that it is normal not to be perfectly happy after a child's birth. If caregivers have serious problems, such as in postnatal depression, you can point out the path to emotional health.

We realize that families come in all varieties. If there is a problem with the baby, all families will behave differently. Your sensitive appreciation of the unique way each family functions can allow you to become a part of the team. Try to notice who gives support to whom, and who suppresses their fears, possibly to their own detriment. Talking to and looking after each member of the family will make you a very welcome and helpful part of the family team.

Treating patients means recognizing their emotional dysfunction and improving it. The most common emotional state of all patients in the hospital is anxiety, even with normal newborns. It comes with the room, no extra charge. One of your most important functions as a doctor is to help relieve that anxiety—nothing that you do as a clinician will be more appreciated. If the child's prognosis is favorable, that should be a pretty easy job, although not in all cases. If the prognosis is unknown or guarded, you can still relieve if not extinguish anxiety, using the techniques described previously.

In dealing with anxiety, framing of the situation is an important technique that has wide use. In what perspective can we put the situation to alleviate anxiety? An example occurred when a young boy needed an atrial septal defect (ASD) repair. His parents found themselves at the university hospital with all the cardiac patients who were to be operated on that week, many with complicated heart lesions that would never be normal. In the midst of more serious disease, his mother said, "Aren't we lucky that it's only an ASD?" Putting a situation in perspective is invaluable in pediatric care. See Table 39.1.

Informing without provoking undue anxiety is an art. It is important not to be dramatic and not to point to the worst possible thing that could happen. An example of what can be said to parents with a newborn that has a high total bilirubin is: "It is a very common condition, one easily treated. We know what causes it and we rarely see problems with it, and if it should unexpectedly get worse, we can always do other procedures to relieve it. So, even though we have to use these lights, and possibly your child will be in the hospital a day or two after you go home, she

Table 39.1 Dealing with anxiety

* Frame the question judiciously
* Do not overly dramatize
* Validate the patient's anxiety
* Listen to patient's conerns

is in no real danger. So you don't really have to worry—even though you will."

If a family does press you to deal with worst-case scenarios, you can then address the problem of their worries directly. Validate their feelings—tell them that you can understand that they would be anxious; were you in their position, you would be anxious yourself.

Your openness can permit the family to talk to you directly about their feelings. Anxiety arises from many sources; the source is different with every family. Their fear may arise from something that happened to a relative, or to a little girl up the street. You can allay their specific fears, but only if you place yourself in a position to discover those fears.

The anxiety of families whose children have mild or transitory illness is more easily relieved than that of seriously ill newborns. Being both truthful and compassionate at the same time is difficult. Your need to relieve the pain of your patients tempts you to reassure them when it is inappropriate; you must tell the truth, if asked. If you have bad news that you must communicate to the patient, be caring, speak simply, and sit down, ready to listen. You can help it hurt a little less by being there with the family and sharing their pain. A practitioner's job is to relieve the patient's distress through all means, not just medicine or surgery.

CARING FOR THE WHOLE PATIENT—INFANT AND PARENTS

Get the newborn the best care possible. This effort not only helps the newborn, but also comforts the family and the practitioner. Also, give the family the best possible care for them: your availability. Tell them you recognize they are under great stress and that they need to take care of themselves along with the newborn. At the same time that you make yourself available, give the family limits ("Call me anytime during the day, when I'll be available at my office."), so that they understand that you won't be much of a doctor unless you get the chance to go home and rest yourself. Encourage the family to seek all possible resources, including friends, neighbors, and community groups. Although lawsuits will still occur, practitioners who have a close relationship with the family reduce their chances of being involved in a suit.

In the past, patients were supposed to trust practitioners without questioning. Power and knowledge were very asymmetric. Now, practitioners are required to inform patients fully about all medical procedures, both legally and ethically. But, information cannot replace the therapeutic value of a human connection. A smile and a soft word are often more important than the latest journal article on the baby's condition.

Both families and practitioners differ in personality and intellectual abilities. A good practitioner knows how much information the patient wants and needs. For some, understanding their child's condition in detail can be a great aid. They feel an increased sense of control with increasing knowledge. Still, all families are able to absorb only a limited amount of information. Especially under stress, repetition will be needed. Likewise, writing things down and using handouts increases retention of information. On the other hand, some families will want to know only the outlines of the case and will want to trust in you. That wish needs to be respected, and force-feeding of information will be counterproductive. They will want to know progress, and they will want to know prognosis; that will be enough.

Appendices

Laboratory Values

Abnormal means more than 2 standard deviations from the mean, not pathologic.

Laboratory values are difficult to assign in the well nursery. Many of the values in the first 24 hours of life represent the mother's condition at birth and not the baby's. For instance, most of the components of the baby's basic metabolic panel (BMP)—electrolytes, serum urea nitrogen (BUN), creatinine—will reflect the mother's blood values for an indeterminate number of hours after birth. Values for other tests such as the prothrombin time (PT) and the activated partial thromboplastin time (PTT) may be extremely high in the first few hours of life without implying any clotting problems.

Because of the small size of newborn samples, technical problems also bedevil obtaining correct laboratory values. If a heelstick required multiple punctures and a great deal of squeezing to obtain an adequate sample, then hemolysis will increase the total bilirubin level by as much as 2 mg/dL. In a 2-day-old child with an actual serum total bilirubin of 8 mg/dL, this can increase the result by 25% and change therapy by engendering an outpatient bilirubin follow-up.

Another example of technical difficulties leading to critically high lab values can be found in the measurement of newborn hematocrits. Heelsticks may change the proportion of serum to plasma in the aliquot drawn. The process of doing a heelstick can change the ratio of serum to plasma by literally squeezing the plasma out of the sample before it is collected. Thus, a hematocrit that by arterial or venous draw would be 58% might initially by heelstick be the critical value of 64%. A basic rule is that, in a stable child, one should do an arterial or venous draw before believing any critical value and acting on it.

The values listed below are the average value of the associated test in multiple laboratories plus or minus two standard deviations from the mean. Unless otherwise marked, these are the values for the first week of life in a full-term infant.

Test	Value CU	Value SI (If Different)	Tissue Source/Comment
Acid phosphatase	13 ± 6 u/L		RBCs
Alanine aminotranferase (ALT)	<45 U/L		Liver/muscle
Albumin	4 ± 1.5 g/dL		Blood
Alkaline phosphatase	280 ± 140 U/L		Tissue breakdown
Ammonia	120 ± 30 mcg/dL	86 ± 22 mcmol/L	Liver—send on ice
Amylase	35 ± 30 U/L		Pancreas/glands
Aspartate aminotransferase (AST)	25 ± 25 U/L		Tissue breakdown
Bicarbonate	20 ± 4 mEq/L		Acid/base metabolyte
Bilirubin—see Chapter 15			1 mg/dL = 17 mcmol/L
Bilirubin, conjugated	<15% of total		RBCs
Arterial blood gas			Make sure arterial sample
At birth			
pH	7.27 ± 0.02		
P_{O_2}	60 ± 5 mmHg		Off oxygen
P_{CO_2}	52 ± 3 mmHg		
After 24 hr			
pH	7.37 ± 0.02		
P_{O_2}	70 ± 5 mmHg		Off oxygen
P_{CO_2}	35 ± 3 mmHg		
BUN (see urea nitrogen)			
Calcium, total	9.0 ± 1.4 mg/dL	2.2 ± 0.4 mmol/L	Full-term only

Calcium, ionized	4.85 ± 0.65 mg/dL	1.2 ± 0.15 mmol/L	1st 2 days/full-term only
Carbon dioxide	18 ± 4 mEq/L	same mmol/L	Full-term only
Chloride	106 ± 8 mEq/L	same mmol/L	Electrolyte
C-reactive protein (CRP)	<0.8 mg/dL		Check specific lab
Creatinine (Phospho) Kinase	105 ± 95 U/L		Muscle/brain
Creatinine	<1 mg/dL	<90 mcmol/L	Protein
Erythrocyte sedimentation (ESR)	<5 mm/hr		Run quickly
Ferritin	110 ± 90 ng/mL		
Fibrinogen	2.3 ± 0.7 g/L		
Folate, serum	35 ± 30 ng/mL	400 ± 60 nmol/L	Must have fed $\times$ 24 hr
Galactose	<20 mg/dL	<1.1 mmol/L	
Gamma glutamyl transferase (GGT)	<130 u/L		
Glucose (see Chapter 7)	>40 mg/dL Day 1	>2.2 nmol/L Day 1	Safe minimum is disputed
Hemoglobin F	$75 \pm 5\%$		Drops rapidly with time
Hemogram			
White blood cells (WBC)	21 ± 12 10^3/mm^3		$<5 \times 10^3$ is a sign of sepsis
Hemoglobin (HB)	16 ± 3.5 g%		
Hematocrit	$51 \pm 9\%$		>60% implies hyperviscosity
Mean corpuscular volume (MCV)	108 ± 10		Check for dysphasic poulation
Platelets (plt)	290 ± 130 10^3/mm^3		$<50 \times 10^3$ is critical value
Reticulocytes (retic)	$5 \pm 2\%$		Elevated in hemolysis
Iron	175 ± 75 mcg/dL	31 ± 13 mcmol/L	
Lactate	<27 mg/dL	<3 mmol/L	

(continued)

Test	Value CU	Value SI (If Different)	Tissue Source/Comment
Lactate dehydrogenase	530 ± 240 U/L		Tissue breakdown
Lead	<3 mcg/dL	<0.15 mcmol/L	Essentially background
Lipase	<90 U/L		
Lipids	<child levels		
Magnesium	1.65 ± 0.35 mE/L	0.85 ± 0.15 mmol/L	↑ when mom on Mg drip
Methemoglobin	<1.5% of Hg		
Osmolality	285 ± 10 mOsm/kg		
Phenylalanine	2.1 ± 1.1 mg/dL	140 ± 65 mcmol/L	Must have fed × 24 hr
Phosporus	6.8 ± 2.2 mg/dL	2.2 ± 0.7 mmol/L	Full-term only
Potassium	4.8 ± 1.1 mEq/L	same mmol/L	Electrolyte
Protein, total	6.0 ± 1.6 g/dL		
PT	13 ± 2.9 sec		Check specific lab
PTT, activated	43 ± 13 sec		Check specific lab
Pyruvate	0.6 ± 0.3 mg/dL	0.065 ± 0.035 mmol/L	
Sodium	140 ± 7 mEq/L	same mmol/L	Electrolyte
SGOT (see AST)			
SGPT (see ALT)			
Transferrin	200 ± 70 mg/dL	same in g/L	
Urea nitrogen (BUN)	8 ± 4 mg/dL	5 ± 3.9 mmol/L	
Uric acid	4.4 ± 2 mg/dL	0.26 ± 0.12 mmol/L	
Zinc	95 ± 25 mcg/dL	14.5 ± 3.8 mcmol/L	

Formulary

Remember to document all medications given to the newborn, including pain medications such as acetaminophen or ibuprofen. Not documenting suggested use of pain medication is a common mistake.

The formulary in this appendix is very limited. It includes only five areas:

1. Medications for the minor problems commonly encountered in the well baby nursery (nystatin)

2. Resuscitation medications that NALS and PALS include in the treatment of apneic and asystolic situations (dopamine or epinephrine)

3. Medications for sepsis or presumed sepsis (antibiotics, antivirals)

4. Medications that a baby might be discharged on if the baby has spent some time in an intensive care nursery before being discharged from the well baby nursery (anti-GERD drugs)

5. Pain medication

For other drugs, the more detailed lists in *The 5-Minute Pediatric Consult* (from which this list is modified) or a general pediatric handbook are suggested.

The medications are listed alphabetically by generic names, but all common U.S. trade names are included in the list with reference to the generic name. Few of the medications listed are actually officially approved in children, let alone newborns, but the doses listed are the generally accepted ones.

PAIN IN THE NEWBORN NURSERY

A special comment must be made about pain medication in the well nursery. Pain in the newborn is a difficult area to quantify. Before 1990, most pediatric references ignored pain in the newborn infant, and unfortunately, so did most practitioners. Until quite recently, the norm for hospital circumcision was no anesthesia at all, not even feeding the newborn sugar water immediately afterward. In many papers over the last

15 years, it has become clear that infants and fetuses probably start to feel pain as early as the second trimester of pregnancy. For both ethical practice and because of the emphasis that licensing authorities, such as the Joint Commission on Accreditation of Hospitals and Medical Organizations, have placed on pain management, it is paramount that the practitioner objectively assess the newborn for pain, document that assessment, and treat the pain found. All three areas have associated difficulties.

Medical organizations and individual practitioners assess pain by using one or more of the many tools that have been documented for childhood pain with NFCS, NIPS, and CREEPS being the most frequently used in the newborn nursery. All of these pain assessment tools have a common problem: they are designed for surgical situations or what one may call "state changes." They are best for comparing changes in discomfort over time rather than seeing if the infant is in pain right now. Therefore, it is best to use the specific tool to determine a baseline so that if a question of pain arises, it can be fairly assessed. To assess pain, we must use observation and an objective scale approved by our hospital or in common use locally. The practitioner can then use that scale to document the pain assessment. Remember that if the assessment is not documented, later observers will assume that the assessment was not done.

Although there are studies that show that opiates relieve severe pain, the proven pain-suppression efficacy of over-the-counter medications such as acetaminophen or ibuprofen in newborns is limited. Both acetaminophen and ibuprofen are antipyretics along with being pain-suppressors. Because fever is a primary sign of sepsis in the first few weeks of life, many practitioners are reluctant to mask this primary manifestation of infection. One must always balance pain relief with the increased risk of missed diagnosis. Non-medication-based pain relief is a practical alternative. Papoosing (wrapping tightly in a blanket), gentle rhythmic motion, and, especially, sucrose water are effective. In fact, in a large meta-analysis combining many different individual research projects, sucrose water was as effective for mild to moderate pain as either acetaminophen or ibuprofen.

Last, the multiple forms of acetaminophen and ibuprofen can easily lead to prescribing errors. The dosage of both medications, which are given in Table A.1, are simple. But distinguishing infant drops from children's liquid is not simple, and distinguishing the more than 10 different-sized chewable pills, tablets, and capsules of each medication is much more difficult. When writing orders, being redundant is good (two 50 mg chewable tablets = 100 mg total), and when giving these medications to new parents, often writing a prescription, even for an over-the-counter drug, is another way to ensure that the correct dose is given.

Medication	Dosage	Comments
Acetaminophen (Tylenol)	Infant drops 80 mg/0.8 mL 10–15 mg/kg/dose PO q6–8hr	Use only when necessary as this interferes with recognition of fevers. Dosage in full-term newborns is usually 0.4 mL
Acyclovir (Zovirax)	IV 50 mg/mL >35 wk gestation 60 mg/kg/24 hr divided q8hr for 21 days	Use routinely in septic infants
Adenosine	IV 3 mg/mL Use PALS algorithm; start with 0.1 mg/kg rapid IV push; if ineffective, go to 0.2 mg/kg IV push 2 min later	Used in PALS protocol for supraventricular tachycardia. Maximum dose 12 mg
Adrenaline—see epinephrine		
Advil—see ibuprofen		
Alprostadil (Prostin VR Pediatric) prostaglandin E	IV 500 mcg/mL Start with 0.05 mcg/kg/min, may increase to max. of 0.2 mcg/kg/min; if effective, decrease immediately to lowest effective dose	To maintain patency of ductus arteriosus in congenital heart disease
Amiodarone HCl (Cordarone)	Use only with cardiac consultation	For pulseless ventricular fibrillation
Ampicillin	IV newborn >2,000 g Sepsis 75 mg/kg/24 hr, meningitis 150 mg/kg/24 hr; both q8hr	Rarely used alone, usually with an aminoglycoside, until organism known

(continued)

Medication	Dosage	Comments
AquaMEPHYTON—see phytonadione		
Ativan—see lorazepam		
Bactroban—see mupirocin cream		
Caffeine	Loading dose 10 mg/kg caffeine base. Maintenance 2.5 mg/kg caffeine base starting 24 hr after loading. Solution and injection both 10 mg/mL.	For apnea. Monitor serum levels daily for first few days
Ceftriaxone (Rocephin)	Not meningitis: 50 to 75 mg/kg/day in 2 doses. Meningitis: 100 mg/kg/day in 1 or 2 doses	Vials from 250 mg to 2 gm. Important to check strength. Reconstitute with lidocaine to minimize pain
Cephalexin (Keflex)	25 to 100 mg/kg/day in 4 doses. Oral suspension 125 or 250/5 mL	Excellent for staph aureus skin infections
Cimetidine (Tagamet)	5 to 10 mg/kg/day in 2 or 3 daily doses. Oral suspension 300 mg/5 mL	
Cordarone—see amiodarone HCl		
Cotazym—see pancrelipase		
Creon—see pancrelipase		
Diastat Rectal—see diazepam		
Diazepam (Diastat Rectal, Valium)	0.05 to 0.3 mg/kg/dose IV or rectal. Rectally 2.5 mg (usually use 1/2 in neonate). IV 5 mg/mL	For status epilepticus
Diazoxide (Hyperstat IV, Proglycem)	Orally 8 mg/kg/day in 2 or 3 doses. May increase slowly to maximum of 15 mg/kg/day. IV 1 to 3 mg/kg every 20 min	For hypertensive emergency

Drug	Dose	Comments
Diflucan—see fluconazole		
Digoxin (Lanoxin)	Total digitalizing dose (TDD): half TDD initially, then 1/4 TDD 8–12 hr later, then 1/4 TDD 8–12 hr after that. Maintenance doses are administered in 2 divided doses beginning 12 hr after the last digitalizing dose. The TDD in a full-term neonate is 25–35 mcg orally or 20–30 mcg IV with oral maintenance 6–10 mcg per day	Must individualize the dose with serum levels prior to next dose to maintain levels of 0.8–2 ng/mL after digitalization. Must monitor with continuous ECG during digitalization
Dilantin—see phenytoin		
Dopamine	2–20 mcg/kg/min IV	For decompensated shock
Edrophonium (Enlon, Reversol, Tensilon)	IV: 0.1 mg, increase by 0.1 to maximum of 0.5 mg	In children with symptoms of myasthenia gravis secondary to in utero exposure
Enlon—see edrophonium		
Epinephrine (Adrenalin)	0.01 to 0.03 mg/kg every 3 to 5 min in trachea. For 3.5 kg, neonate dose is 1 c of 1:10,000 solution	For cardiac arrest
Ergocalciferol	400 units per day in healthy children. 1,000 units per day in malabsorption syndromes	Give if family history of vitamin D disorders. Massive doses up to 500,000 units per day in familial vitamin D resistant rickets—consult endocrinology
Erythromycin ophthalmic ointment	Apply 0.5% ointment TID to both eyes	Use in staph aureus conjunctivitis

(continued)

229

Medication	Dosage	Comments
Feverall—see acetaminophen		
Fluconazole (Diflucan)	6 mg/kg day 1, then 3 mg/kg for 14 days. If child under 14 days of age, usually given in same doses but every 48 hr	Resistant oral candidiasis
Folic acid (Folvite, vitamin B6)	25 to 35 mcg daily RDA. To replace in deficiency, 15 mcg/kg/day	For megaloblastic anemias
Folvite—see folic acid		
Furosemide (Lasix)	1 to 2 mg/kg/dose q6–12 hr	Management of fluid balance in congested heart failure
Garamycin—see gentamycin		
Gentamycin	Full-term 2.5 mg/kg every 8–12 hr	Follow with peak and trough values
Gentamycin ophthalmic drops	0.3% OU TID 2–3 drops	Conjunctivitis
Glucose	IV through large vein 0.5 to 1 g/kg, which is equivalent to 10–20 mL/kg of 5% glucose; 5–10 mL/kg of 10% glucose; 2–4 mL/kg of 25% glucose	Give slow IV or IO push
Glucagon	Neonates 0.025 mg/kg/dose parenterally	Care of hypoglycemia not responding to oral or IV glucose
Hydrocotisone ointment/cream	1% and $2\frac{1}{2}$% available	Use for significant eczema and contact reaction
Hydrocortisone oral	Congenital adrenal hyperplasia: initially 30–36 mg/kg/day divided as 1/3 in the morning and 2/3 in the evening or 1/4 in the morning, 1/4 midday, and 1/2 in the evening. Oral suspension 10 mg/5 mL	Maintenance 0.5–0.75 mg/kg/day

Hyperstat IV—see diazoxide		
Ibuprofen (Advil, Motrin, Nuprin)	Oral dose is 10 mg/kg q6hr. Liquid 100 mg/5 mL, drops 40 mg/mL	See section on neonatal pain
Inderal—see propanolol		
Indocin—see indomethacin		
Indomethacin	Use in intensive care situation only. Initial 0.2 mg/kg/dose is followed by 2 doses based on patient's postnatal age (PNA) at time of first dose: PNA < 48 hours: 0.1 mg/kg at 12–24-hr intervals; PNA 2–7 days: 0.2 mg/kg at 12–24-hr intervals; PNA > 7 days: 0.25 mg/kg at 12–24-hr intervals	Nonsurgical closure of patent ductus. The patient's renal and hepatic function should be monitored
INH—see isoniazid		
Insulin	Regular insulin loading dose of 0.1 unit/kg followed by continuous 0.1/kg/hr	Rarely used in neonate unless total pancreatic failure
Isoniazid (INH)	9 mg/kg/day. Recommendations for course length are varied. Minimum of 3 mo	Pyridoxine may be needed in breast-fed infants. See Table in Appendix C or consult *Red Book* for details
Keflex—see cephalexin		
Lanoxin—see digoxin		
Lasix—see furosemide		
Levothyroxine (Levothroid, Synthroid)	8–10 mcg/kg/day. Tablets start at 25 mcg	Usually not started until metabolic screen reported back from state

(continued)

231

Medication	Dosage	Comments
Lidocaine	For cardiac arrhythmias: 1 mg/kg loading dose, followed by a continuous 20–50 mcg/kg/min	Also used by infiltration for local anesthesia. Maximum dose 4.5 mg/dose and at least 2 hr between doses
Lorazepam (Ativan)	0.05 mg/kg parenterally over 2–5 min. May repeat in 15 min	For status epilepticus
Magnesium sulfate	25–50 mg/kg IV or IO over 10–20 min	
Metoclopramide (Reglan)	0.1–0.5 mg/kg/day in 4 divided doses before meals; 0.8 mg/kg/day maximum	For gastroesophageal reflux
Motrin—see ibuprofen		
Mupirocin (Bactroban) cream	Apply TID for 5 days	For infected superficial wounds
Mycostatin—see nystatin		
Nafcillin	Parenteral 60 mg/kg/24 hr in 4 to 6 doses	Nonresistant staph aureus infections
Naloxone (Narcan)	0.01 mg/kg parenterally every 2 to 3 min if depressed from neonatal opiate depression. Endotracheal dose is 0.1 mg/kg	Endotracheal dose may have delayed onset of action. May be necessary to redose every 1–2 hr (infants have poor glomerular filtration rates and may maintain high doses of opiates for prolonged periods of time)
Narcan—see naloxone		
Nembutol—see phenobarbital		
Neostigmine (Prostigmin)	0.04 mg/kg single dose	For myasthenia gravis test

Drug	Dose	Comments
Nilstat—see nystatin		
Nuprin—see ibuprofen		
Nystatin (Mycostatin, Nilstat)	Thrush: 2 mL of oral suspension rubbed around mouth QID—60 mL bottle with dropper. Diaper dermatitis: apply cream TID, 15 and 30 g tubes	
Omeprazole (Prilosec)	0.6 to 1.0 mg/kg/dose, usually once daily	In hypersecretory cases, may give BID
Palivizumab (Synagis)	15 mg/kg/mo IM	Use in RSV
Pancrease MT—see Pancrelipase		
Pancrelipase (Cotazym, Creon, Pancrease MT, Zymase)	2,000 to 4,000 lipase units per 4 oz of formula (120 mL)	Used in known cystic fibrosis patients
Penicillin G, aqueous	Neonates under age 7 days: <2,000 g: 25,000 U/kg every 12 hr. For meningitis, use 50,000 U/kg every 12 hr. >2,000 g: 20,000 U/kg every 8 hr. For meningitis, 50,000 U/kg every 8 hr. Neonates over age 7 days: <2,000 g: 25,000 U/kg every 8 hr. For meningitis, 50,000 U/kg every 8 hr. >2,000 g: 25,000 U/kg every 6 hr. For meningitis, 50,000 U/kg every 6 hr	Available as both K+ and NA+ salts. Only drug proven for treatment of syphylis. Benzathine penicillin is not recommended in newborns, because it may lead to sterile abscesses and procaine toxicity

(continued)

233

Medication	Dosage	Comments
Phenobarbital (Nembutal)	Loading dose 15–20 mg/kg PO or parenteral with 3–5 mg/kg/day maintenance dose given BID	Therapeutic serum range is 15–40 mcg/mL
Phenytoin (Dilantin)	Loading dose 15–20 mg/kg PO or parenteral. Maintenance dose 5–8 mg/kg/day BID or TID	Therapeutic serum range is 8–15 mcg/mL in neonates
Phytonadione (vitamin K, AquaMEPHYTON)	0.5–1 mg within 1 hr of birth IM	Oral administration of IM dose might work, but there is no definitive data. Written consent should be obtained if parents refuse IM or insist on oral administration
Prilosec—see omeprazole		
Proglycem—see diazoxide		
Propranolol (Inderal)	2 mg/kg/day for thyrotoxicosis orally	May also be used for arrhythmias and tetralogy of Fallot spells rarely
Propylthiouracil	5–10 mg/kg/day TID	Once hyperthyroid symptoms are gone, may use lower dose (113 of initial treatment)
Prostigmin—see neostigmine		
Prostin VR Pediatric—see alprostadil		
Ranitidine (Zantac)	2–4 mg/kg/day BID orally	Some children need much higher dosage to control high acid levels
Reglan—see metoclopramide		

Drug	Dose	Notes
Reversol—see edrophonium		
Rocephin—see ceftriaxone		
Tagamet—see cimetidine		
Tempra—see acetaminophen		
Tensilon—see edrophonium		
Tylenol—see acetaminophen		
Sodium bicarbonate	1 mEq/kg/dose IV	Use only under intensivist consultation. May lead to brain swelling and subsequent brain damage
Synagis—see palivizumab		
Valium—see diazepam		
Vanocin—see vancomycin		
Vancomycin (Vancocin)	For neonates under age 7 days: <1,000 g: 10 mg/kg every 24 hr. 1,000–2,000 g: 10 mg/kg every 18 hr. >2,000 g: 10 mg/kg every 12 hr	For treatment of methicillin-resistant staph aureus
Vitamin B6—see folic acid		
Vitamin D—see ergocalciferol		
Vitamin K—see phytonadione		
Zantac—see ranitidine		
Zidovudine	See Chapter 12 for details	
Zovirax—see acyclovir		
Zymase—see pancrelipase		

SUGGESTED READING

Schwartz MW, ed. *5-minute pediatric consult,* 3th ed. Philadelphia: Lippincott Williams & Wilkins, 2003.

APPENDIX C
Breast Feeding and Medications

Unfortunately, the lack of knowledge we have about which materials are dangerous in breast milk in vast. To the best possible knowledge in 2003, the following list is up-to-date.

The following cautions are:
A – Completely safe
B – Probably completely safe
C – Use with mild caution
D – Use if no alternative exists
X – Do *not* use

Drug	Risk Factor Category	Effect While Breast Feeding
Acetazolamide	C	Compatible
Acetohexamide	D	Data not available
Acetophenazine	C	Data not available
Acetylcholine	C	Data not available
Acyclovir	C	Compatible
Adenosine	C	Data not available
Albuterol	C	Data not available
Alfentanil	C (D with prolonged use)	Clinical significance probably nil
Allopurinol	C	Compatible
Alphaprodine	C (D with prolonged use)	Data not available
Alprazolam	D	Causes lethargy and irritability
Amantadine	C	Use with caution
Ambenonium	C	Compatible
Amikacin	C	Use with caution
Aminocaproic acid	C	Data not available
Aminoglutethimide	D	Data not available
Aminophylline	C	Compatible
Aminopterin	X	Data not available
para-Amino-salicylic acid	C	Inconclusive
Amiodarone	C	Not recommended
Amitriptyline	D	Unknown but of concern
Amlodipine	C	Data not available
Amobarbital	D	Data not available
Amoxapine	C	Unknown but of concern
Amphetamine	C	Contraindicated
Amrinone	C	Data not available
Amyl nitrite	C	Data not available
Anileridine	D with prolonged use	Data not available
Anisindione	D	See coumarin derivatives

(continued)

Drug	Risk Factor Category	Effect While Breast Feeding
Anisotropine	C	Compatible
Antazoline	C	Data not available
Aprobarbital	C	Data not available
Aprotinin	C	Data not available
Asparaginase	C	Data not available
Aspirin	C (D if in 3rd trimester)	Use with caution
Atenolol	C	Compatible
Atropine	C	Compatible
Aurothioglucose	C	See gold sodium thiomalate
Azathioprine	D	Data not available
Bacitracin	C	Data not available
Baclofen	C	Compatible
Beclomethasone	C	See prednisone
Belladonna	C	See atropine
Benazepril	D	See captopril
Bendroflumethiazide	D	Suppresses lactation (chlorothiazide)
Benzthiazide	D	See chlorothiazide
Benztropine	C	See atropine
Bepridil	C	Data not available
Betacarotene	C	Data not available
Betamethasone	C	Data not available
Betaxolol	C	May cause hypotension, bradycardia
Bethanechol	C	Abdominal pain and diarrhea in infant
Biperiden	C	See atropine
Bismuth subsalicylate	C	Use with caution
Bisoprolol	C	May cause hypotension, bradycardia
Bleomycin	D	Data not available
Bretylium	C	Data not available
Bromides	D	Compatible
Bromocriptine	C	Contraindicated
Bromodiphenhydramine	C	Data not available
Brompheniramine	C	Compatible usually
Buclizine	C	Data not available
Bumetanide	D	Diuretic, may suppress lactation
Busulfan	D	Data not available
Butalbital	C (D with prolonged use)	See pentobarbital
Butaperazine	C	Data not available
Butoconazole	C	Data not available
Butorphanol	D with prolonged use	Compatible

(continued)

238

Drug	Risk Factor Category	Effect While Breast Feeding
Camphor	C	Data not available
Captopril	D	Compatible
Carbachol	C	Data not available
Carbamazepine	C	Compatible
Carbarsone	D	Data not available
Carbimazole	D	See methimazole
Carbinoxamine	C	Data not available
Carphenazine	C	Data not available
Carteolol	C	May cause hypotension, bradycardia
Casanthranol	C	See cascara sagrada
Cascara sagrada	C	Compatible
Chenodiol	X	Data not available
Chloral hydrate	C	Compatible
Chlorambucil	D	Data not available
Chloramphenicol	C	Not recommended
Chlorcyclizine	C	Data not available
Chlordiazepoxide	D	See diazepam
Chloroquine	C	Compatible
Chlorothiazide	D	Compatible, may suppress lactation
Chlorotrianisene	X	See oral contraceptives
Chlorpromazine	C	Unknown but of concern
Chlorpropamide	D	Data not available
Chlorprothixene	C	Unknown but of concern
Chlortetracycline	D	Compatible
Chlorthalidone	D	See chlorothiazide
Chlozoxazone	C	Data not available
Cholestyramine	C	Data not available
Ciguatoxin	X	Not recommended
Cinnarizine	C	Data not available
Ciprofloxacin	C	Not recommended
Cisplatin	D	Compatible
Clemastine	C	Use with caution
Clidinium	C	Compatible
Clofazimine	C	Causes hyperpigmentation in infant
Clofibrate	C	Data not available
Clomiphene	X	Data not available
Clomipramine	C	Compatible
Clomocycline	D	See tetracycline
Clonazepam	C	May cause CNS depression or apnea
Clonidine	C	May cause hypotension

(continued)

239

Drug	Risk Factor Category	Effect While Breast Feeding
Clorazepate	D	Unknown but of concern
Cocaine	C (X if nonmedicinal use)	Contraindicated
Codeine	C (D with prolonged use)	Compatible
Colchicine	D	Compatible
Corticotropin/ cosyntropin	C	Data not available
Cortisone	D	Data not available
Coumarin derivatives	D	Phenindione is contraindicated and warfarin and dicumarol are compatible
Cyclamate	C	Data not available
Cyclandelate	C	Data not available
Cyclazocine	D	Data not available
Cyclopenthiazide	D	See chlorothiazide
Cyclophosphamide	D	Contraindicated
Cycloserine	C	Compatible
Cyclosporine	C	Contraindicated
Cyclothiazide	D	See chlorothiazide
Cycrimine	C	See atropine
Cytarabine	D	Data not available
Dacarbazine	C	Data not available
Dactinomycin	C	Data not available
Danazol	X	Data not available
Danthron	C	See cascara sagrada
Dantrolene	C	Data not available
Daunorubicin	D	Data not available
Decamethonium	C	Data not available
Deferoxamine	C	Data not available
Demecarium	C	Data not available
Demeclocycline	D	See tetracycline
Desipramine	C	Unknown but of concern
Deslanoside	C	See digitalis
Dexamethasone	C	Data not available
Dexbrompheniramine	C	See brompheniramine
Dextroamphetamine	C	See amphetamine
Dextrothyroxine	C	Data not available
Diatrizoate	D	See potassium iodide
Diazepam	D	Unknown but of concern
Diazoxide	C	Data not available
Dibenzepin	D	See imipramine
Dichlorphenamide	C	Data not available

(*continued*)

Drug	Risk Factor Category	Effect While Breast Feeding
Dicoumarol	D	See coumarin derivatives
Dienestrol	X	May decrease milk production and decrease nitrogen and protein content
Diethylstilbestrol	X	May decrease milk production and decrease nitrogen and protein content
Diflunisal	C (D in 3rd trimester)	Data not available
Digitalis	C	Compatible
Digitoxin	C	See digitalis
Digoxin	C	See digitalis
Diltiazem	C	Compatible
Dimethindene	C	Data not available
Dimethothiazine	C	Data not available
Dioxyline	C	Data not available
Diphemanil	C	See atropine
Diphenadione	D	See coumarin derivatives
Diphenhydramine	C	Contraindicated
Diphenoxylate	C	Compatible
Dipyridamole	C	No known problems
Disopyramide	C	Compatible
Disulfiram	C	Data not available
Dobutamine	C	Data not available
Docusate calcium	C	Data not available
Docusate potassium	C	Data not available
Docusate sodium	C	Diarrhea in infant
Dopamine	C	Data not available
Dothiepin	D	Unknown but of concern
Doxepin	C	Unknown but of concern
Doxorubicin	D	Contraindicated
Doxycycline	D	Compatible
Droperidol	C	Data not available
Dyphylline	C	Compatible
Echothiophate	C	Data not available
Edrophonium	C	Compatible
Electricity	D	Data not available
Enalapril	D	Compatible
Ephedrine	C	Causes irritability in infant
Epinephrine	C	Data not available
Epoetin Alfa	C	Data not available
Ergotamine	D	Contraindicated

(continued)

Drug	Risk Factor Category	Effect While Breast Feeding
Erythrityl tetranitrate	C	Data not available
Esmolol	C	Data not available
Estradiol	X	Compatible
Estrogens, conjugated	X	See mestranol, ethinyl estradiol
Estrone	X	See estrogens, conjugated
Ethacrynic acid	D	Contraindicated
Ethanol	D (X if used for long periods)	Use with caution
Ethchlorvynol	C	Data not available
Ethinamate	C	Data not available
Ethinyl estradiol	X	May decrease milk production and decrease nitrogen and protein content
Ethiodized oil	D	See potassium iodide
Ethisterone	D	See oral contraceptives
Ethoheptazine	C	Data not available
Ethopropazine	C	See atropine
Ethosuximide	C	Compatible
Ethotoin	D	Data not available
Ethyl biscoumacetate	D	See coumarin derivatives
Ethynodiol	D	See oral contraceptives
Etretinate	X	Contraindicated
Evans blue	C	Data not available
Felodipine	C	Data not available
Fenfluramine	C	Data not available
Flecainide	C	Compatible
Flosequinan	C	Data not available
Fluconazole	C	Probably safe
Flucytosine	C	Data not available
Flunitrazepam	D	Unknown, probably insignificant
Fluorouracil	D	Data not available
Flupenthixol	C	Unknown but of concern
Fluphenazine	C	See prochlorperazine
Flurazepam	X	Unknown but of concern
Folic acid	C if used in excess	Compatible
Fosinopril	D	See captopril and enalapril
Furazolidone	C	Data not available

(*continued*)

Drug	Risk Factor Category	Effect While Breast Feeding
Furosemide	C	See chlorothiazide
Gadopentetate dimeglumine	C	Data not available
Gentamicin	C	Could cause bloody stool
Gentian violet	C	Data not available
Gitalin	C	See digitalis
Glyburide	D	Data not available
Glycerin	C	Data not available
Gold sodium thiomalate	C	Compatible
Griseofulvin	C	Data not available
Guaifenesin	C	Data not available
Guanabenz	C	Data not available
Haloperidol	C	Unknown but of concern
Heparin	C	Compatible
Heroin	D if used in excess	Contraindicated
Hexachlorophene	C	Use in nipple washing may
Hexamethonium	C	Data not available
Hexocyclium	C	See atropine
Homatropine	C	See atropine
Hormonal pregnancy test tablets	X	See oral contraceptives
Hydralazine	C	Compatible
Hydriodic acid	D	See potassium iodide
Hydrochlorothiazide	D	See chlorothiazide
Hydrocodone	D if used in excess	Data not available
Hydroflumethiazide	D	See chlorothiazide
Hydromorphone	D if used in excess	Data not available
Hydroxychloroquine	C	Compatible
Hydroxyprogesterone	D	Data not available
hydroxyurea	D	Contraindicated
Hydroxyzine	C	Data not available
I-Hyoscyamine	C	See atropine
Hyperalimentation, parenteral	C	Compatible
Ibuprofen	D if used in 3rd trimester	Compatible
Idoxuridine	C	Data not available
Imipramine	D	Unknown but of concern
Immune globulin, intramuscular	C	Data not available
Immune globulin, intravenous	C	Data not available
Immune globulin, hepatitis B	C	Data not available

(continued)

Drug	Risk Factor Category	Effect While Breast Feeding
Immune globulin, rabies	C	Data not available
Immune globulin, tetanus	C	Data not available
Immune globulin, varicella-zoster (human)	C	Data not available
Indapamide	D	Data not available
Iocetamic acid	D	See potassium iodide
Iodinated glycerol	X	See potassium iodide
Iodine	D	See potassium iodide
Iodipamide	D	See potassium iodide
Iodoquinol	C	Data not available
Iodoxamate	D	See potassium iodide
Iopanoic acid	D	Compatible
Iothalamate	D	See potassium iodide
Ipodate	D	See potassium iodide
Iprindole	D	See imipramine
Iproniazid	C	See phenelzine
Isocarboxazid	C	Data not available
Isoetharine	C	Data not available
Isoflurophate	C	Data not available
Isoniazid	C	Compatible
Isopropamide	C	See atropine
Isoproterenol	C	Data not available
Isosorbide	C	Data not available
Isosorbide dinitrate	C	Data not available
Isosorbide mononitrate	C	Data not available
Isotretinoin	X	See vitamin A
Isoxsuprine	C	Data not available
Isradipine	C	Data not available
Kanamycin	D	Compatible
Kaolin/pectin	C	Compatible
Ketoconazole	C	Data not available
Ketoprofen	D if used in 3rd trimester	Compatible
Labetalol	C	Compatible
Laetrile	C	Data not available
Lanatoside C	C	See digitalis
Leucovorin	C	See folic acid
Leuprolide	X	Data not available
Levallorphan	D	Data not available
Levarterenol	D	Data not available
Levorphanol	D if used for long periods	Data not available
Lidocaine	C	Compatible
Lipids	C	Data not available
Lisinopril	D	See captopril and enalapril

(*continued*)

Drug	Risk Factor Category	Effect While Breast Feeding
Lithium	D	Containdicated
Lorazepam	D	Unknown but of concern
Lovastatin	X	Unknown but of concern
Loxapine	C	Data not available
Lynestrenol	D	See oral contraceptives
Lypressin	C	See vasopressin
Lysergic acid diethylamide (LSD)	C	Unknown but of concern
I-Lysine	C	Data not available
Mandelic acid	C	Imconclusive
Mannitol	C	Data not available
Marijuana	C	Contraindicated
Mazindol	C	Data not available
Mebanazine	C	See phenelzine
Mebendazole	C	Compatible
Mechlorethamine	D	Data not available
Meclofenamate	D if used in 3rd trimester	Data not available
Medroxyproges- terone	D	Compatible
Mefloquine	C	Data not available
Melphalan	D	Data not available
Menadione	C (X if used near delivery)	See phytonadione
Mepenzolate	C	See atropine
Meperidine	D if used for long periods	Compatible
Mephentermine	C	Data not available
Mephenytoin	C	Data not available
Mephobarbital	D	See phenobarbital
Mepindolol	C	Data not available
Meprobamate	D	Data not available
Mercaptopurine	D	Data not available
Mesoridazine	C	Unknown but of concern
Mestranol	X	See oral contraceptives
Metaproterenol	C	Data not available
Metaraminol	D	Data not available
Methacycline	D	See tetracycline
Methadone	D if used for long periods	Compatible
Methamphetamine	C	See amphetamine
Methantheline	C	See atropine
Methaqualone	D	Data not available
Metharbital	D	Data not available
Methazolamide	C	Data not available
Methdilazine	C	Data not available

(*continued*)

Drug	Risk Factor Category	Effect While Breast Feeding
Methenamine	C	Compatible
Methimazole	D	Compatible
Methixene	C	See atropine
Methocarbamol	C	Compatible
Methotrexate	D	Contraindicated
Methotrimeprazine	C	Data not available
Methoxamine	C	Data not available
Methscopolamine	C	See atropine
Methsuximide	C	Data not available
Methyclothiazide	D	See chlorothiazide
Methyldopa	C	Compatible
Methylene blue	C	Data not available
Methylphenidate	C	Data not available
Metolazone	D	See chlorothiazide
Metrizamide	D	Compatible
Metrizoate	D	See potassium iodide
Mexiletine	C	Compatible
Miconazole	C	Data not available
Midazolam	D	Data not available
Mifepristone	X	Contraindicated
Milrinone	C	Data not available
Mineral oil	C	Data not available
Minocycline	D	See tetracycline
Minoxidil	C	Compatible
Misoprostol	X	Contraindicated
Molindone	C	Data not available
Morphine	D if used for long periods	Compatible
Moxalactam	C	Compatible
Nadolol	C	Compatible
Nalbuphine	D if used for long periods	Data not available
Nalorphine	D	Data not available
Naproxen	D if used in 3rd trimester	Compatible
Neomycin	C	Data not available
Neostigmine	C	See pyridostigmine
Niacin	A (C if used in excess)	See niacinamide
Niacinamide	A (C if used in excess)	Compatible
Nialamide	C	Data not available
Nicardipine	C	Data not available
Nicotinyl alcohol	C	Data not available
Nicoumalone	D	See coumarin derivatives
Nifedipine	C	Compatible
Nimodipine	C	Data not available
Nitroglycerin	C	Data not available
Nizatidine	C	Compatible
Nonoxynol-9/ octoxynol-9	C	Data not available

(*continued*)

Drug	Risk Factor Category	Effect While Breast Feeding
Norethindrone	X	Compatible
Norethynodrel	X	Compatible
Norgestrel	X	See oral contraceptives
Nortriptyline	D	Unknown but of concern
Novobiocin	C	Unknown but of concern
Nutmeg	C	Data not available
Nylidrin	C	Data not available
Oleandomycin	C	Data not available
Olsalazine	C	See mesalamine
Omeprazole	C	Data not available
Opipramol	D	See imipramine
Opium	D if used for long periods	See morphine
Oral contraceptives	X	Compatible under close supervision
Orphenadrine	C	See atropine
Oxazepam	D	See diazepam
Oxprenolol	C	Compatible
Oxtriphylline	C	See theophylline
Oxycodone	D if used for long periods	Data not available
Oxymetazoline	C	Data not available
Oxymorphone	D if used for long periods	Data not available
Oxyphenbutazone	D	See phenylbutazone
Oxyphencyclimine	C	See atropine
Oxyphenonium	C	See atropine
Oxytetracycline	D	See tetracycline
Pantothenic acid	C if used in excess	Compatible
Paramethadione	D	Data not available
Paregoric	D if used for long periods	See morphine
Pargyline	C	Data not available
Paromycin	C	Data not available
Penbutolol	C	Data not available
Penicillamine	D	Contraindicated
Pentaerythritol tetranitrate	C	Data not available
Pentamidine	C	Data not available
Pentazocine	D if used for long periods	Data not available
Pentobarbital	D	Data not available
Pentoxifylline	C	Inconclusive
Perphenazine	C	Unknown but of concern
Phenazocine	D if used for long periods	Data not available
Phencyclidine	X	Contraindicated
Phendimetrazine	C	Data not available
Phenelzine	C	Data not available

(continued)

Drug	Risk Factor Category	Effect While Breast Feeding
Phenindione	D	See coumarin derivatives
Pheniramine	C	Data not available
Phenobarbital	D	Use with caution
Phenolphthalein	C	Data not available
Phenoxybenzamine	C	Data not available
Phenprocoumon	D	See coumarin derivatives
Phensuximide	D	Data not available
Phentermine	C	See amphetamine
Phentolamine	C	Data not available
Phenylbutazone	C (D if used in 3rd trimester)	Compatible
Phenylephrine	C	Data not available
Phenylpropanolamine	C	Data not available
Phenyltolaxamine	C	Data not available
Phenytoin	D	Compatible
Physostigmine	C	Data not available
Phytonadione	C	Compatible
Pilocarpine	C	Data not available
Piperacetazine	C	Compatible
Piperidolate	C	See atropine
Piroxicam	D if used in 3rd trimester	Compatible
Plicamycin	D	Data not available
Polythiazide	D	See chlorothiazide
Potassium iodide	D	Compatible
Povidone iodine	D	See potassium iodide
Prazosin	C	Data not available
Primaquine	C	Data not available
Primidone	D	Use with caution
Procainamide	C	Compatible
Procarbazine	D	Data not available
Prochlorperazine	C	Compatible
Procyclidine	C	See atropine
Promazine	C	Data not available
Promethazine	C	Data not available
Propafenone	C	Data not available
Propantheline	C	See atropine
Propoxyphene	C (D if used for long periods)	Compatible
Propranolol	C	Compatible
Propylthiouracil	D	Compatible
Protamine	C	Data not available
Protirelin	C	See levothyroxine
Protriptyline	C	Data not available
Pseudoephedrine	C	Compatible
Pyrantel pamoate	C	Data not available
Pyrazinamide	C	Data not available

(continued)

Drug	Risk Factor Category	Effect While Breast Feeding
Pyrethrins with piperonyl butoxide	C	Data not available
Pyridostigmine	C	Compatible
Pyidoxine	C if used in excess	Compatible
Pyrilamine	C	Data not available
Pyrimethamine	C	Compatible
Pyrvinium pamoate	C	Data not available
Quinacrine	C	Data not available
Quinapril	D	See captopril
Quinethazone	D	See chlorothiazide
Quinidine	C	Compatible
Quinine	D	Compatible
Ramipril	D	See captopril
Reserpine	C	Data not available
Ribavirin	X	Data not available
Rifampin	C	Compatible
Saccharin	C	Compatible
Scopolamine	C	Compatible
Secobarbital	D	Compatible
Senna	C	Compatible
Simethicone	C	Data not available
Sodium iodide	D	See potassium iodide
Sodium iodide (125)	X	See sodium iodide (131)
Sodium iodide (131)	X	Contraindicated
Sodium nitroprusside	C	Data not available
Spiramycin	C	Data not available
Spironolactone	D	Compatible
Streptokinase	C	Data not available
Streptomycin	D	Compatible
Sulfasalazine	D if used near term	Use with caution
Sulfonamides	D if used near term	Compatible
Sulindac	D if used in 3rd trimester	Data not available
Temazepam	X	Unknown but of concern
Teniposide	D	Data not available
Teraxosin	C	Data not available
Terconazole	C	Data not available
Terfenadine	C	Data not available
Tetanus/diphtheria toxoids (adult)	C	Data not available
Tetrabenazine	C	Data not available
Tetracycline	D	Compatible
Theophylline	C	Compatible
Thiabendazole	C	Data not available
Thioguanine	D	Data not available
Thiopropazate	C	Data not available
Thioridazine	C	Data not available

(*continued*)

Drug	Risk Factor Category	Effect While Breast Feeding
Thiotepa	D	Data not available
Thiothixene	C	Data not available
Thiphenamil	C	See atropine
Thyrotropin	C	Data not available
Timolol	C	Compatible
Tobramycin	C	Data not available
Tocainide	C	Data not available
Tolazamide	D	Data not available
Tolazoline	C	Data not available
Tolbutamide	D	Compatible
Tolmetin	C (D if used near delivery)	Compatible
Tranylcypromine	C	Data not available
Trazodone	C	Unknown but of concern
Triamterene	D	Data not available
Triazolam	X	Data not available
Trichlomethiazide	D	See chlorothiazide
Tridihexethyl	C	See atropine
Trientine	C	Data not available
Trifluoperazine	C	Data not available
Triflupromazine	C	Data not available
Trihexyphenidyl	C	See atropine
Trimeprazine	C	Compatible
Trimethadione	D	Data not available
Trimethaphan	C	Data not available
Trimethobenzamide	C	Data not available
Trimethoprim	C	Compatible
Triprolidine	C	Compatible
Troleandomycin	C	See oleandomycin
Tyropanoate	D	See potassium iodide
Urea	C	Data not available
Valproic acid	D	Compatible
Vancomycin	C	Data not available
Verapamil	C	Compatible
Vidarabine	C	Data not available
Vinblastine	D	Data not available
Vincristine	D	Data not available
Warfarin	D	See coumarin derivatives
Zidovudine	C	Data not available
Zuclopenthixol	C	Use with caution

(continued)

Vaccines	Risk Factor Category	Effect While Breast Feeding
BCG	C	Data not available
Cholera	C	Data not available
E. coli	C	Data not available
Hemophilus B conjugate	C	Data not available
Hepatitis B	C	Data not available
Influenza	C	Compatible
Measles	X	Data not available
Mumps	X	Data not available
Plague	C	Data not available
Pneumococcal polyvalent	C	Data not available
Poliovirus inactivated	C	Data not available
Poliovirus live	C	Avoid before 6 wk
Rabies (human)	C	Data not available
Rubella	X	No adverse effects
Smallpox	X	Data not available
Tularemia	C	Data not available
Typhoid	C	Data not available
Yellow fever	D	Data not available

Online Resources

Online resources change constantly. Some are not updated regularly. Some are abandoned entirely, but still stay on the Internet. Some require payment to get into or are limited to members only. Some of the best free sites as of this writing (December 2003) and a book on how to access them are listed below.

- Dover GJ, McMillan MD. *Pediatrics and Neonatology: An Internet Resource Guide*. Montvale, NJ: Thomson Medical Economics, 2003.

  One of the most stable and continuously updated sites is:

- KidsHealth: *http://www.kidshealth.org/*

I am employed by the Nemours Foundation, which built and maintains this site, but I would still recommend it first if I did not work for them. Links for patients and professionals.
   Other stable sites are:

- Eat Smart Play Hard: http://www/fns.usda.gov/eatsmartplayhard/
  A wonderful site for children (and their parents) to learn about nutrition.

- Nutrition and Your Child: http://www.bcm.tmc.edu/cnrc.
  This enables you to find other resources on the Internet. For instance, the breast-feeding site has all the links to published documents one would need, including all the policy statements of major organizations and of the self-help groups such as La Leche.

- National Center for Education in Maternal and Child Health: *http://www.ncemch.org*
  Huge data base prescreened on the topic of nutrition in mothers and children.

- United States Maternal and Child Health Bureau: *http://www.mchb.hrsa.gov/default.htm*
  Again, mainly a guide to other sources with a good link to Bright Futures.

- Bright Futures: *http://brightfutures.aap.org/web/SearchResults.asp*
  A great source for anticipatory guidance.

Index

Note: Page numbers followed by *f* indicate figures; page numbers followed by *t* indicate tables.